Compensating for Quasi-periodic Motion in Robotic Radiosurgery

Floris Ernst

Compensating for Quasi-periodic Motion in Robotic Radiosurgery

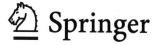 Springer

Floris Ernst
Institute for Robotics and Cognitive Systems
University of Lübeck
Lübeck, Germany

ISBN 978-1-4899-9528-5   ISBN 978-1-4614-1912-9 (eBook)
DOI 10.1007/978-1-4614-1912-9
Springer New York Dordrecht Heidelberg London

Printed on acid-free paper

Springer is part of Springer Science+Business Media (www.springer.com)

Web resources

In this work, several scripts for MATLAB as well as data sets for evaluation and a motion prediction toolkit have been introduced. All these items are available for public download from `http://signals.rob.uni-luebeck.de`.

Contents

Acknowledgements

I would like to express my gratitude towards my supervisor, Prof. Dr.-Ing. Achim Schweikard, who gave me the opportunity to work on this highly fascinating topic. I am much indebted to him for allowing me to freely pursue my ideas and for always providing support. I also thank Prof. Dr. rer. nat. Bernd Fischer, my thesis' second referee, for his valuable input.

I would also like to thank my colleagues—I really enjoyed working with you. I would especially like to mention Lars Matthäus, Ralf Bruder, and Alexander Schlaefer for their help with unfamiliar topics, for proof reading my work and for the time they spent working with me on my experiments. Parts of my work would not have been possible without the assistance of my students, especially the work of Matthias Knöpke and Norman Rzezovski should be acknowledged here. And, of course, the heart and soul of our institute, Cornelia Rieckhoff, must be mentioned: she was always willing to help with the difficulties of the English language, the pitfalls of working at the university, and the minor and major organisational and personal problems that came up during my time here.

Last but not least I express my gratitude towards my family, my parents, and my friends for their support and for reading my work for clarity, spelling and grammar.

Curriculum Vitae

Floris Ernst was born on August 6th, 1981, in Hinsdale, Illinois/USA. He studied Mathematics at Friedrich-Alexander-University (Erlangen, Germany) and at the University of Otago (Dunedin, New Zealand).

He graduated from the University of Otago in 2004 with a Postgraduate Diploma in Sciences (Mathematics). In 2006, he graduated From Friedrich-Alexander-University with a Diploma in Mathematics, minoring in Computer Sciences.

From 2006 on he held a position as a research associate at the University of Lübeck's Institute for Robotics and Cognitive Systems, where he worked on motion compensation strategies in robotic radiosurgery. He graduated from this university with a Ph.D in 2011.

Chapter 1
Introduction

Interest in motion compensation in radiotherapy was sparked in the 1990s, when a new device for intracranial radiosurgery, the CyberKnife®, was invented. This machine, described in more detail in section 2.2, makes use of a standard industrial robot carrying a light-weight linear accelerator. While, at first, it was solely intended for stereotactic treatment of intracranial tumours, it has been extended to be the world's first system capable of compensating respiratory motion in radiotherapy. For the first time, this system allowed the creation and delivery of highly conformal treatment plans for moving tumours, i.e., it became possible to precisely irradiate a moving tumour with a high dose while sparing adjacent healthy tissue. Clearly, this is only possible if both the location of the tumour is known at any time and the delivery system can compensate for this motion in real time.

These two main issues, however, have not been fully solved yet. It is not yet possible to locate the target region in real time without exposing the patient to too much additional radiation. Compensating for systematic latencies, which arise from data acquisition, signal processing, and mechanical inertia, is also an active field of research.

1.1 The Problem of Latency

One of the problems arising in robotic radiosurgery is the fact that motion of a mechanical device following human motion (i.e., respiration or pulsation) cannot be instantaneous. Latencies occur inevitably in the signal processing chain and the robot control system. A schematic overview of possible sources of latencies is given in figure 1.1.

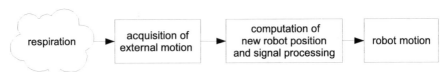

Fig. 1.1: Sources of latency

Sources of Latency

The amount of latency accrued from each step in figure 1.1 varies greatly: current tracking systems operate at very high frequencies and latencies of around 10 ms are common. The time needed for the second step, determination of the new robot position, is strongly dependent on the computations needed. Typically, this will involve inverse kinematics of the robot, determination of the tumour position from the surrogate signal, and the time needed for motion prediction. In total, this may take anywhere from less than 1 ms to 20 ms, depending on the algorithms employed. We will address this issue later. The third and most relevant source of latency comes from the robotic system itself: due to mechanical constraints, it cannot move instantaneously but requires some time for acceleration and deceleration. Currently used systems exhibit robotic delays of approximately 75 to 100 ms. In total, we will have to deal with a latency of approximately 100 to 150 ms, which has to be compensated by prediction. The issue of predicting respiratory or pulsatory motion will be addressed in chapter 4, the correlation model between external surrogates and tumour motion will be covered in chapter 5.
Another source of latency is caused by the patient's anatomy. Depending on the type, location, and shape of the tumour as well as the patient's general condition and breathing behaviour, there may be a significant phase shift between the motion of the tumour and the motion as recorded using external surrogates. This phase shift has been examined in great detail, and delays of up to 200 ms have been reported [17, 32, 34]. This latency, however, cannot be compensated for by prediction, since it is not known a priori. Its compensation must be incorporated into the correlation model relating external to internal motion.

Latencies of Motion Compensation Systems

Multiple motion tracking and compensation systems have been described in literature, ranging from open-loop control systems like Accuray's CyberKnife, BrainLAB's VERO, TomoTherapy's MAD, and multiple DMLC approaches, to closed-loop control systems where the treatment couch is moved. Of these systems, only the CyberKnife is currently used in the clinic, the VERO system is available clinically, but—until now—without the motion compensation component. All other devices are currently research-only. The systematic latencies of these systems, however, have been described in literature. They range from under 50 ms for the VERO system [9] to more than second using a couch compensation method [12]. The current generation of the CyberKnife has a latency of about 115 ms [31], down from 192.5 ms in the previous version [15], which is still widely in use. The DMLC or SMART approaches, using different MLCs, have latencies from approximately 150 ms to 570 ms [4–8, 18, 21, 24–26, 28–30, 33, 36, 38] due to different tracking modalities used (EM, kV X-ray, MV X-ray, optical, or combinations thereof). The approaches moving the treatment couch have delays from about 300 ms to more than one second [12, 14, 23, 35, 39]. An overview is given in figure 1.2.

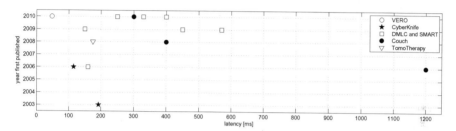

Fig. 1.2: Latencies of different motion compensation devices. Data from [4–9, 12, 14, 15, 18, 21–26, 28–31, 33, 35, 36, 38, 39]

Table 1.1: Components of the latency of a system based on a Varian MLC (kV tracking), the VERO, TomoTherapy MAD, and CyberKnife systems. Data from [9, 11, 19, 22, 27].

	VERO	MLC	MAD	CyberKnife
position acquisition	25 ms	309 ms[a]	30 ms	25 ms[d]
position calculation	2 ms	20 ms	—	15 ms[d]
gimbals/MLC/robot control cycle	20 ms	52 ms	45 ms	75 ms[d]
other	—	38 ms[b]	100 ms[c]	—
total	47 ms	420 ms	175 ms	115 ms

[a] This figure includes the time needed to write the kV image to disk and an (unknown) delay before the image is actually written. The authors of [27] suspect it to be approximately 95 % of the imaging sampling distance, in this case 140 ms (6.67 Hz imaging frequency).
[b] This is the time needed to read the kV image from disk.
[c] By design, the TomoTherapy machine delivers one projection every 200 ms, so 100 ms must be added to the system's latency [22].
[d] These numbers are approximate, from [19].

These latencies are combined latencies, i.e., the sum of latencies from different sources. While in most cases the individual components of the latency are unknown, for the VERO system [9], one of the Varian MLC systems [27], the TomoTherapy MAD approach [22], and the current generation CyberKnife [19], we know the individual components. They are given in table 1.1.

Note that in this table all but the MLC-based systems use some form of optical tracking to detect the target position. From [27] we know that the kV imaging method used in MLC tracking is very slow, and that—due to flaws in the current design—it should be possible to reduce the actual latency to about 170 ms. If other 3D localisation methods would be used, like 3D ultrasound, stereoscopic X-ray imaging, or MV imaging, the position acquisition latencies would be approximately 30-45 ms for ultrasound tracking (see section 5.2.2.1), 100 ms for X-ray localisation [9], and 270 ms [27] for MV imaging.

1.2 Medical Background

In 2008, about 216,000 people died from malign neoplasms (ICD-10 C00 to C97) in Germany, corresponding to 25.6 % of all deaths in this year [10]. This makes cancer the most prevalent cause of death for middle-aged people and the second most common cause of death in the general population, surpassed only by cardiovascular disease (see figure 1.3).

Although both diagnosis and therapy of tumours has become more advanced in recent years, the share of deaths from malign neoplasms in Germany has stayed relatively constant. Over the years 2002 to 2008, it ranges from 24.5 % (2003) to 25.7 % (2006) with a mean of 25.4 % [10]. This clearly shows the necessity of improving care for cancer patients. For the U.S., similar data exist [37]: in 2007, the leading cause of death was cardiovascular disease, accounting for about 806,000 deaths (33.3 %), malign neoplasms, as the second-most prevalent cause of death, accounted for about 563,000 deaths (23.2 %).[1]

What we can see from the data collected in Germany, however, is the fact that the mean age at which cancer patients die is increasing, it has gone up from 70.27 years in 2002 to 71.36 years in 2008, figure 1.4. This shows that the survival time of cancer victims is rising but patients still die from their cancer.

Apart from surgery and chemotherapy, radiotherapy is the method of choice for curative or palliative treatment of many neoplasms, especially for lung cancer [3]. We now focus on solid tumours in organs that strongly move with respiration, like the thoracic organs and certain alimetary organs (like the liver, the pancreas, or the kidneys). For these organs, a problem which has only been targeted in the past fifteen years [20] becomes obvious: the tumour will also move with respiration, making it harder to treat with radiotherapy. A closer look at figure 1.3 reveals that the second largest group of deaths from malign neoplasms is caused by cancer of thoracic organs. That these tumours are indeed hard to cure is confirmed by table 1.2, which shows the trends in five year survival rates of liver, pancreatic and lung/bronchus cancer in the U.S.. We can see that they all are very aggressive and that the chance of surviving these cancers has only slightly increased in the past 35 years.

---

[1] Both the data from Germany [10] and the data from the U.S. [37] include deaths from malign neoplasms of lymphoid, hematopoietic and related tissue (ICD-10 codes C81 to C96), which can clearly not be treated by radiosurgery (around 17,000 deaths in Germany in 2008 and around 55,000 deaths in the U.S. in 2007).

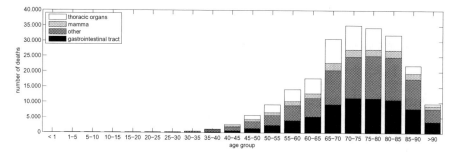

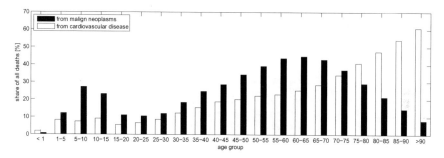

Fig. 1.3: Deaths from malign neoplasms in Germany in 2008. The top graph shows the absolute number of deaths per age group, the bottom graph shows the share of all deaths for malign neoplasms and cardiovascular disease. Numbers taken from [10].

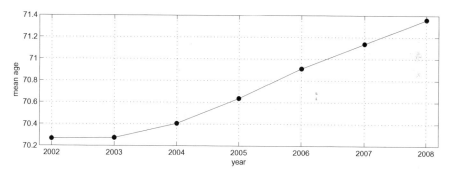

Fig. 1.4: Mean age of cancer victims aged 1 to 90 years in Germany, 2002 to 2008 (numbers computed using data taken from [10]).

Given these numbers, it is clear that treatment tumours moving with respiration is one of the most rewarding fields: radiotherapeutic treatment can benefit tremendously from improved target tracking and localisation methods, which have become feasible only recently.

Table 1.2: Trends in 5-year Relative Survival Rates* (%) by Race and Year of Diagnosis, U.S., 1975-2004 (reproduced with permission from "American Cancer Society. *Cancer Facts and Figures 2009*. Atlanta: American Cancer Society, Inc." [2])

Site	All races 1975-77	1984-86	1996-2004	White 1975-77	1984-86	1996-2004	African American 1975-77	1984-86	1996-2004
All sites	50	54	66†	51	55	68†	40	41	58†
Brain	24	29	35†	23	28	34†	27	33	39†
Breast (female)	75	79	89†	76	80	91†	62	65	78†
Colon	52	59	65†	52	60	66†	46	50	55†
Esophagus	5	10	17†	6	11	18†	3	8	11†
Hodgkin lymphoma	74	79	86†	74	80	87†	71	75	80†
Kidney	51	56	67†	51	56	67†	50	54	66†
Larynx	67	66	64†	67	68	66	59	53	50
Leukemia	35	42	51†	36	43	52†	34	34	42
Liver‡	4	6	11†	4	6	10†	2	5	8†
Lung & bronchus	13	13	16†	13	14	16†	11	11	13†
Melanoma of the skin	82	87	92†	82	87	92†	60§	70§	78
Myeloma	26	29	35†	25	27	35†	31	32	33
Non-Hodgkin lymphoma	48	53	65†	48	54	66†	49	48	58
Oral cavity	53	55	60†	55	57	62†	36	36	42†
Ovary	37	40	46†	37	39	45†	43	41	38
Pancreas	3	3	5†	3	3	5†	2	5	5†
Prostate	69	76	99†	70	77	99†	61	66	96†
Rectum	49	57	67†	49	58	67†	45	46	59†
Stomach	16	18	25†	15	18	23†	16	20	25†
Testis	83	93	96†	83	93	96†	82‡	87‡	87
Thyroid	93	94	97†	93	94	97†	91	90	95
Urinary bladder	74	78	81†	75	79	82†	51	61	66†
Uterine cervix	70	68	73†	71	70	74†	65	58	65
Uterine corpus	88	84	84†	89	85	86†	61	58	61

* Survival rates are adjusted for normal life expectancy and are based on cases diagnosed in the SEER 9 areas from 1975-1977, 1984-1986, and 1996-2004, and followed through 2005. † The difference in rates between 1975-1977 and 1996-2004 is statistically significant (p <0.05). ‡ The standard error of the survival rate is between 5 and 10 percentage points. § The standard error of the survival rate is greater than 10 percentage points. # Includes intrahepatic bile duct.

1.3 Purpose of this Work

The aim of this work is to improve the algorithmical basis of cancer treatment in the presence of quasi-periodic motion. This is achieved by looking at methods to predict the time series stemming from human respiratory and pulsatory motion as well as looking into ways of computing the target region's motion based on sparse internal data and frequent external measurements. These two issues are the core of this work, which has been performed within the framework of the DFG research project Schw 502/8-3, a part of the SPP 1124 (Schwerpunktprogramm, priority programme) Medizinische Navigation und Robotik (robotics and navigation in medicine).

More specifically, the goal is to analyse methods already used in the clinic and compare them, using an unprecedented amount of test data, to newly developed algorithms. In this context, special focus was placed on a common framework for prediction algorithms to allow for simple inclusion of new methods.

Additionally, the use of one single error measure, the RMS error, as an indicator of prediction or correlation quality, is questioned. Since the distribution and "randomness" of the error is important in the context of radiotherapy, new ideas to base quality assessment on other measures were examined.

1.4 Organisation

This work is structured as follows: in chapter 2, the medical consequences of moving targets in radiotherapy are described and the basic principles of motion compensated radiosurgery are explained. State of the art treatment methods are presented and radiosurgical systems currently in use are described. Additionally, a new application of radiosurgery, treating atrial fibrillation, is outlined.

Chapter 3 starts with two experiments. In the first experiment, the systematic latencies of an optical tracking device are determined. In the second experiment, the latencies of an open control loop where a robot follows the motion of an optical marker are measured. The chapter then focuses on new techniques to determine the accuracy of motion prediction and correlation and on ways to improve the signal-to-noise ratio of respiratory or pulsatory motion traces. The measures introduced are based on the distance between the true motion and the predicted motion, on the velocity occuring in the predicted motion trace, and on the regularity of the error. The noise reduction method presented makes use of Wavelet decomposition and is specifically tailored to real-time processing of quasi-periodic signals sampled at high frequencies. The last part of chapter 3 is geared towards reducing artefacts from tracking active infrared markers.

In chapter 4, seven prediction algorithms are introduced. One method, called EKF, is based on Extended Kalman Filtering and relies on the assumption that human respiratory motion can be represented as a superposition of finitely many sinusoidals (section 4.1). Four algorithms, the nLMS, FLA-nLMS, RLS, and wLMS algorithms, are based on the idea that respiration is a stationary process (sections 4.2.1 and 4.2.2). The MULIN algorithm (section 4.2.3) exploits the fact that respiratory signals are close to being piecewise linear, and the SVRpred algorithm (section 4.2.4) tries to model prediction as a high dimensional regressor in kernel space. Three of these algorithms, the MULIN, wLMS, and FLA-nLMS algorithms, have been newly developed in this work. Two further algorithms, the EKF and SVRpred algorithms, are based on known principles which have, for the first time, been expanded and adapted to respiratory motion prediction. The remaining two algorithms, the nLMS and RLS algorithms, are slightly modified versions of well-known methods. Furthermore, the influence of the novel noise reduction method (presented in section 3.3) on prediction quality is evaluated in section 4.3. A prediction toolkit is introduced and the algorithms are evaluated on a database of 304 respiratory motion traces.

Chapter 5 then deals with the problem of computing the position of an internal target region based on motion traces recorded on the patient's chest or abdomen. The algorithms in clinical use and a new algorithm based on Support Vector Regression are explained in section 5.1. The algorithms are validated in an animal study using implanted gold fiducials and in a volunteer study using 3D ultrasound of the liver.

Finally, chapter 6 gives an overview of the results, discusses possible standards for signal processing, and proposes to establish a publicly available database of motion traces.

References

[1] American Association of Physicists in Medicine: Annual Meeting of the AAPM, vol. 52 (2010)

[2] American Cancer Society: Cancer Facts & Figures. American Cancer Society, Atlanta (2009)

[3] Belderbos, J., Sonke, J.J.: State-of-the-art lung cancer radiation therapy. Expert Review of Anticancer Therapy **9**(10), 1353–1363 (2009). DOI 10.1586/era.09.118

[4] Ceberg, S., Falk, M., af Rosenschöld, P.M., Gustafsson, H., Korreman, S., Bäck, S.: Tumor-tracking radiotherapy of a moving target during arc delivery: verification using polymer gel and a diode array. In: ESTRO 29 [13], p. S74

[5] Cho, B.C., Poulsen, P.R., Ruan, D., Sawant, A., Povzner, S., Keall, P.J.: DMLC tracking with real-time target position estimation combining a single kV imager and an optical respiratory monitoring system. International Journal of Radiation Oncology, Biology, Physics **75**(3, supp.), S24–S25 (2009)

[6] Cho, B.C., Poulsen, P.R., Sawant, A., Ruan, D., Keall, P.J.: Real-time target position estimation using stereoscopic kilovoltage/megavoltage imaging and external respiratory monitoring for dynamic multileaf collimator tracking. International Journal of Radiation Oncology, Biology, Physics p. in press (2010). DOI 10.1016/j.ijrobp.2010.02.052

[7] Cho, B.C., Poulsen, P.R., Sloutsky, A., Sawant, A., Keall, P.J.: First demonstration of combined kV/MV image-guided real-time dynamic multileaf-collimator target tracking. International Journal of Radiation Oncology, Biology, Physics **74**(3), 859–867 (2009). DOI 10.1016/j.ijrobp.2009.02.012

[8] Cho, B.C., Suh, Y., Dieterich, S., Keall, P.J.: A monoscopic method for real-time tumour tracking using combined occasional X-ray imaging and continuous respiratory monitoring. Physics in Medicine and Biology **53**(11), 2837–2855 (2008). DOI 10.1088/0031-9155/53/11/006

[9] Depuydt, T., Haas, O.C.L., Verellen, D., Erbel, S., de Ridder, M., Storme, G.: Geometric accuracy evaluation of the new VERO stereotactic body radiation therapy system. In: UKACC International Conference on CONTROL 2010, vol. 8, pp. 259–264. United Kingdom Automatic Control Council, Coventry, UK (2010)

[10] DEStatis: Todesursachen in Deutschland 2002–2008, *Fachserie 12 – Gesundheitswesen*, vol. 4. Statistisches Bundesamt Wiesbaden (2004–2010). URL http://www.destatis.de

[11] Dieterich, S.: Private communication (Mar., 2008, and Oct., 2010)

[12] D'Souza, W.D., McAvoy, T.J.: An analysis of the treatment couch and control system dynamics for respiration-induced motion compensation. Medical Physics **33**(12), 4701–4709 (2006). DOI 10.1118/1.2372218

[13] European Society for Therapeutic Radiology and Oncology: Annual Meeting of the ESTRO, vol. 29 (2010)

[14] Haas, O.C.L.: Motion prediction for predictive couch motion control. In: RT-MART Workshop 2009 [16]

[15] Hoogeman, M., Prévost, J.B., Nuyttens, J., Pöll, J., Levendag, P., Heijmen, B.: Clinical accuracy of the respiratory tumor tracking system of the CyberKnife: Assessment by analysis of log files. International Journal of Radiation Oncology, Biology, Physics **74**(1), 297–303 (2009). DOI 10.1016/j.ijrobp.2008.12.041

[16] Institute for Robotics, University of Lübeck: Real-Time Motion Adaptive Radiation Therapy Workshop 2009 (2009)

[17] Kanoulas, E., Aslam, J.A., Sharp, G.C., Berbeco, R.I., Nishioka, S., Shirato, H., Jiang, S.B.: Derivation of the tumor position from external respiratory surrogates with periodical updating of the internal/external correlation. Physics in Medicine and Biology **52**(17), 5443–5456 (2007). DOI 10.1088/0031-9155/52/17/023

[18] Keall, P.J., Sawant, A., Cho, B.C., Ruan, D., Wu, J., Poulsen, P.R., Petersen, J., Newell, L.J., Cattell, H., Korreman, S.: Electromagnetic-guided dynamic multileaf collimator tracking enables motion management for intensity-modulated arc therapy. International Journal of Radiation Oncology, Biology, Physics **79**(1), 312–320 (2011). DOI 10.1016/j.ijrobp.2010.03.011

[19] Kilby, W.: Accuray, Inc. Private communication (Sep., 2009, and Oct., 2010)

[20] Kubo, H.D., Hill, B.C.: Respiration gated radiotherapy treatment: a technical study. Physics in Medicine and Biology **41**(1), 83 (1996). DOI 10.1088/0031-9155/41/1/007

[21] Larsson, T., Falk, M., Aznar, M., Keall, P.J., Korreman, S., Munck af Rosenschöld, P.: Accuracy of MLC-tracking for inversely optimized arc therapy delivery to moving targets for two different MLCs. In: ESTRO 29 [13], p. S21

[22] Lu, W.: Real-time motion-adaptive delivery (MAD) using binary MLC: II. Rotational beam (tomotherapy) delivery. Physics in Medicine and Biology **53**(22), 6513–6531 (2008)

[23] Malinowski, K.T., Yousuf, M.A., McAvoy, T.J., D'Souza, W.D.: The concept of couch motion compensation. In: RTMART Workshop 2009 [16]

[24] Poulsen, P.R., Cho, B.C., Keall, P.J.: Real-time prostate trajectory estimation with a single imager in arc radiotherapy: a simulation stud. Physics in Medicine and Biology **54**(13), 4019–4035 (2009). DOI 10.1088/0031-9155/54/13/005

[25] Poulsen, P.R., Cho, B.C., Sawant, A., Keall, P.J.: Time analysis of image-based dynamic MLC tracking. In: 51st Annual Meeting of the AAPM, *Medical Physics*, vol. 36, p. 2674. American Association of Physicists in Medicine, Anaheim, CA, USA (2009). DOI 10.1118/1.3182146. SU-FF-T-648

[26] Poulsen, P.R., Cho, B.C., Sawant, A., Keall, P.J.: Implementation of a new method for dynamic multileaf collimator tracking of prostate motion in arc radiotherapy using a single kV imager. International Journal of Radiation Oncology, Biology, Physics **76**(3), 914–923 (2010). DOI 10.1016/j.ijrobp.2009.06.073

[27] Poulsen, P.R., Cho, B.C., Sawant, A., Ruan, D., Keall, P.J.: Detailed analysis of latencies in image-based dynamic MLC tracking. Medical Physics **37**(9), 4998–5005 (2010). DOI 10.1118/1.3480504

[28] Poulsen, P.R., Cho, B.C., Sawant, A., Ruan, D., Keall, P.J.: Dynamic MLC tracking of moving targets with a single kV imager for 3D conformal and IMRT treatments. Acta Oncologica **49**(7), 1092–1100 (2010). DOI 10.3109/0284186x.2010.498438

[29] Sawant, A., Smith, R.L., Venkat, R.B., Santanam, L., Cho, B.C., Poulsen, P.R., Cattell, H., Newell, L.J., Parikh, P.J., Keall, P.J.: Toward submillimeter accuracy in the management of intrafraction motion: the integration of real-time internal position monitoring and multileaf collimator target tracking. International Journal of Radiation Oncology, Biology, Physics **74**(2), 575–582 (2009). DOI 10.1016/j.ijrobp.2008.12.057

[30] Sawant, A., Venkat, R.B., Srivastava, V., Carlson, D., Povzner, S., Cattell, H., Keall, P.J.: Management of three-dimensional intrafraction motion through real-time DMLC tracking. Medical Physics **35**(5), 2050–2061 (2008). DOI 10.1118/1.2905355

[31] Sayeh, S., Wang, J., Main, W.T., Kilby, W., Maurer Jr., C.R.: Robotic Radiosurgery. Treating Tumors that Move with Respiration, 1st edn., chap. Respiratory motion tracking for robotic radiosurgery, pp. 15–30. Springer, Berlin (2007). DOI 10.1007/978-3-540-69886-9

[32] Shirato, H., Seppenwoolde, Y., Kitamura, K., Onimura, R., Shimizu, S.: Intrafractional tumor motion: Lung and liver. Seminars in Radiation Oncology **14**(1), 10–18 (2004)

[33] Smith, R.L., Sawant, A., Santanam, L., Venkat, R.B., Newell, L.J., Cho, B.C., Poulsen, P.R., Cattell, H., Keall, P.J., Parikh, P.J.: Integration of real-time internal electromagnetic position monitoringcoupled with dynamic multileaf collimator tracking: an intensity-modulated radiation therapy feasibility study. International Journal of Radiation Oncology, Biology, Physics **74**(3), 868–875 (2009). DOI 10.1016/j.ijrobp.2009.01.031

[34] Suh, Y., Dieterich, S., Cho, B.C., Keall, P.J.: An analysis of thoracic and abdominal tumour motion for stereotactic body radiotherapy patients. Physics in Medicine and Biology **53**(13), 3623–3640 (2008). DOI 10.1088/0031-9155/53/13/016

[35] Wilbert, J., Meyer, J., Baier, K., Guckenberger, M., Herrmann, C., Hess, R., Janka, C., Ma, L., Mersebach, T., Richter, A., Roth, M., Schilling, K., Flentje, M.: Tumor tracking and motion compensation with an adaptive tumor tracking system (ATTS): system description and prototype testing. Medical Physics **35**(9), 3911–3921 (2008). DOI 10.1118/1.2964090

[36] Wu, J., Ruan, D., Cho, B.C., Sawant, A., Petersen, J., Newell, L.J., Cattell, H., Keall, P.J.: Electromagnetic detection and real-time DMLC correction of rotation during radiotherapy. In: 52nd Annual Meeting of the AAPM [1], p. 3149. DOI 10.1118/1.3468243. SU-GG-J-19

[37] Xu, J., Kochanek, K.D., Murphy, S.L., Tejada-Vera, B.: Deaths: Final data for 2007. National Vital Statistics Report **58**(19) (2010)

[38] Xu, J., Papanikolaou, N., Shi, C., Jiang, S.B.: Synchronized moving aperture radiation therapy (SMART): superimposing tumor motion on IMRT MLC leaf

sequences under realistic delivery conditions. Physics in Medicine and Biology **54**(16), 4993–5007 (2009). DOI 10.1088/0031-9155/54/16/010

[39] Yousuf, M.A., Malinowski, K.T., McAvoy, T.J., D'Souza, W.D.: A novel treatment couch for real-time tracking of respiration induced target motion: Evaluating its geometric accuracy. In: 52nd Annual Meeting of the AAPM [1], p. 3185. DOI 10.1118/1.3468393. SU-GG-T-08

Chapter 2
Motion Compensation in Robotic Radiosurgery

This chapter describes the principles of motion compensation in radiotherapy with a focus on robotic radiosurgery, starting with a brief description of the medical implications. Throughout, special emphasis will be placed on the CyberKnife® system and we will outline the problems originating from the aim of real-time motion compensation. The main current application of robotic radiotherapy is the treatment of malignant tumours while a second, very promising field is the therapy of cardiac arrhythmia, especially of atrial fibrillation. An outline of this project called *CyberHeart*, and the challenges emanating from it, will be given in section 2.5.

2.1 Medical Implications

As a fully automatic system designed to compensate for respiratory and pulsatory motion as well as for motion of the patient, the CyberKnife (and also the CyberHeart extension) allows for treatment of cancerous regions anywhere in the body. Especially important, due to the system's possible sub-millimetre accuracy [19, 48], the treatment of previously inoperable or surgically complex tumours has become possible, opening up a new treatment option for a great multitude of patients.

The aforementioned problem of latency, however, as well as the notoriously difficult task of determining organ motion using non-invasive imaging methods, is responsible for the remaining inaccuracies and limitations of the system. Especially in those cases where tumour motion is large (i.e. tumours in the central lung or tumours close to the diaphragm) and respiration of the patient is irregular, targeting accuracy might be compromised. Consider the situation depicted in figure 2.1: the clinician determines the cancerous area to be treated (called Gross Tumour Volume (GTV)). This area is expanded to include regions where the cancer might have already spread to, i.e., regions where some cells are cancerous. This is called the Clinical Target Volume (CTV), which is further enlarged to cover imaging and treatment uncertainties (then called Planning Target Volume (PTV)). Usually, certain areas of the body are classified as Organ at Risk (OAR), i.e. regions which should be spared from irradiation as much as possible. If planning of the radiosurgical treatment is done at one phase of respiration (e.g. on a breath-hold Computed Tomography (CT) scan) and the treatment is delivered while the patient is breathing freely, the treatment beams might not be placed as planned (figure 2.1).

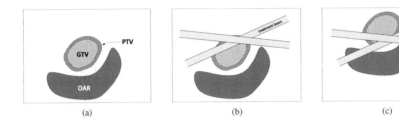

(a)   (b)   (c)

Fig. 2.1: (a) Typical situation of an Organ at Risk (OAR), the Gross Tumour Volume (GTV) and the Planning Target Volume (PTV) (b) Two treatment beams are shown during one respiratory phase (c) The same treatment beams can hit the OAR during another respiratory phase or might miss the GTV

As a consequence, the PTV is usually selected much larger than clinically required to cope with these inaccuracies. Clearly, this artificial enlargement as well as the inevitable blurring of the dose gradients due to organ motion render certain tumours intreatable without motion compensation. Subsequently, when the OARs are too close to the GTV, the enhanced margin required for Conformal Radiation Therapy (CRT), 3D Conformal Radiation Therapy (3DCRT) and other approaches not compensating for motion, can cause severe difficulties when creating the treatment plan. These difficulties can even be so grave that accurate planning and treatment is not possible, not because the GTV cannot be dealt with, but because the OARs would be in too great danger.

2.2 Active Tumour Tracking in Image-Guided Radiotherapy

2.2.1 The CyberKnife

The first system intended to accurately treat tumours anywhere in the human body has been developed from 1987 on by Dr. John R. Adler, Jr., at Stanford University. It was envisioned in [15, 16], initially called *ADLR* [2] and then *Neurotron 1000* [5, 32] and intended for stereotactic radiosurgery of brain tumours. It was first used clinically on June 8, 1994 [3, 63]. The system was subsequently renamed CyberKnife and has been further improved by a collaboration of American and German scientists [4, 6, 7, 10, 41–47]. The system has since been manufactured commercially by Accuray, Inc.,(A) and received U.S. Food and Drug Administration (FDA) approval for treatment of stationary tumours (head, neck and upper spine) in 1999

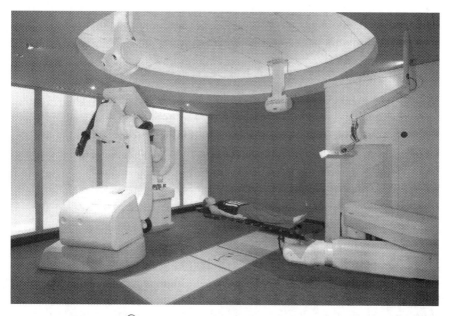

Fig. 2.2: The CyberKnife® (copyright Accuray, Inc.). The figure shows the robotic arm (left) carrying the linear accelerator, the ceiling-mounted X-ray sources, the X-ray detectors (the flat panel on the room's floor), the optical tracking device (ceiling-mounted, on the right) and a patient equipped with the Synchrony® vest on the robotic couch.

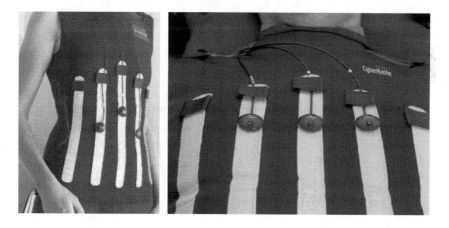

Fig. 2.3: Vest with Synchrony® markers (copyright Accuray, Inc.). Note that the markers can be placed nearly anywhere on the patient's chest.

and for all other body parts in 2001. The system also allows for irradiation of tumours which move with respiration by compensating for this motion. The so-called Synchrony® respiratory tracking system was approved by the FDA in 2004. The current generation of the CyberKnife is shown in figure 2.2.

The system consists of a standard six-jointed industrial robot, the medical version of the KUKA KR 240[(B)], which carries a lightweight Linear Accelerator (LINAC) to generate the treatment beam. The robot is used to position the LINAC at multiple positions around the patient to ensure homogeneous coverage of the tumour with steep dose gradients. Furthermore, the robotic system allows for near real-time compensation of target motion.

The general concept of the CyberKnife is to

- manually delineate tumours in a pre-operative CT scan, to
- create a treatment plan, then to
- match the CT to the position of the patient during treatment, and
- update and correct the positioning to ensure accurate delivery of the prescription dose [62].

The target's position is determined using stereoscopic X-ray imaging of either bony structures [35], clearly visible tumours [45], or artificial landmarks [44], so-called *fiducials*. Typically, the fiducials are gold rods of 3-5 mm length and 0.5-2 mm diameter. In the case of breath-dependent tumours, an external surrogate signal is used to fill the gaps between the acquisition of X-ray shots, wich are taken at irregular intervals, to minimise the radiation dose from imaging. This signal is acquired at approximately 27 Hz with the FlashPoint 5500 (Stryker, Inc.[(C)]) tracking system capable of detecting optical markers. These optical markers are placed on the patient's chest and allow for precise tracking of respiratory motion. A typical setup is shown in figure 2.3.

The procedure of treating breath-dependent tumours can be described as follows:

- The tumour is localised and delineated on a pre-treatment CT scan. In certain cases, fiducials are implanted under CT guidance.
- The patient is placed on the treatment couch and, using stereoscopic X-ray imaging, is registered to the CT scan.
- A correlation model relating the surrogate signal (optical markers on the patient's chest) to the tumour motion is built using several X-ray images.
- The LINAC is placed on predetermined positions to deliver the required radiation dose to the tumour.
- Motion of the patient is monitored by optical tracking and automatically compensated by moving the LINAC. The validity of the correlation model between optical marker motion and tumour motion is checked regularly and the model is updated accordingly.

Figure 2.4 shows a sketch of the principles of robotic radiosurgery. It is important to note that internal organ motion will not be the same as external motion.

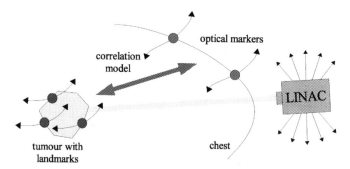

Fig. 2.4: This figure shows the prinicples of robotic radiosurgery, i.e., the moving target, the markers on the patient's chest, the moving LINAC and the correlation model.

2.2.2 Other Approaches

In contrast to moving the LINAC with a robotic arm, two other methods to actively compensate for tumour motion have been devised recently. One is based on moving the patient with a robotised treatment couch [11, 12, 65], the second is based on moving the LINAC using a gimbals approach [18, 22, 60]. The couch method has, until today, not reached clinical practice, whereas the gimbals approach has just been started to be manufactured commercially by Mitsubishi Heavy Industries Medical Systems, Inc.,[D] as MHI-TM2000. It is distributed outside Japan by Brain-LAB AG[E] as the VERO High Precision Radiation Therapy System. It is based on a gimbaled X-ray head and C-band LINAC, both mounted in an O-ring. Using the gimbals mount, the LINAC can easily be moved in two Degrees of Freedom (DOF), the other two relevant DOFs are realised by rotating the O-ring or by skewing the O-ring around its base. Additionally, the patient is set up by means of a motorised couch and the beam can be shaped using a Multi-Leaf Collimator (MLC). The device is shown in figure 2.5. To date, the MHI-TM2000 system has been installed at two Japanese and one overseas site (Brussels University Hospital) [34] where it went operational on 27.11.2009 [61].

Two other methods, which do not directly move the beam source, are also currently under development. The first involves dynamic adaptation of the treatment beam's shape during irradiation. This method, known as Dynamic Multi-Leaf Collimator (DMLC) [24, 30, 31, 38] or Synchronised Moving Aperture Radiation Therapy (SMART) [36, 67], will be covered in section 2.3. The other method tries to incorporate motion information into the delivery of tomotherapy treatment plans, a method called Motion-Adaptive Delivery (MAD). Tomotherapy devices are also described in section 2.4.

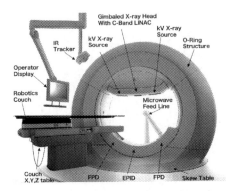

Fig. 2.5: MHI-TM2000 (photograph courtesy of Yuichiro Kamino, MHI Ltd., Tokyo, Japan)

2.3 Gantry-Based Systems

In contrast to robotic systems actively compensating for motion, like the CyberK-nife, or the new O-ring based MHI-TM2000/VERO system, most commonly used radiotherapy devices are gantry-based. This means that the LINAC cannot move in four or more DOFs, but is mounted on a cylindrical assembly in the bore of which the patient is placed. Figure 2.6 shows two different gantry-based systems, being the Elekta[F] Synergy® S, figure 2.6a, and the Varian[G] Clinac, figure 2.6b, systems. These systems usually only allow for rotation around their major axis while patient setup has to be done manually or using a motorised couch.

2.3.1 Respiratory Gating

The usual approach for gantry-based systems is to only irradiate the tumour during certain respiratory phases, e.g. during maximum exhalation. This method is called *gating*. One of the first approaches to monitoring the motion of the target was Mitsu-bishi's Real-Time Respiratory Tracking (RTRT) system. It is a gantry-based system using up to four room-mounted X-ray detectors to track the motion of fiducials im-planted into the tumor. It has been first presented in 1999 [54] and more detailed descriptions were given in 2000 [52, 53]. The RTRT system is shown in figure 2.8. This system, however, did not find wide acceptance, possibly due to the constant additional radiation from fluoroscopic tracking. Although this additional dose is not very high [51], it still seems to be a concern for most physicians, even more so since other, less invasive gating methods are commercially available. One such method is Varian's Real-time Position Management System (RPM), which tracks the chest of a patient using an optical tracking system and an acrylic box with six markers (see figure 2.7a). BrainLAB's ExacTrac® Adaptive Gating method works in a similar

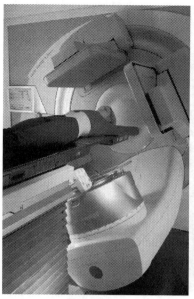
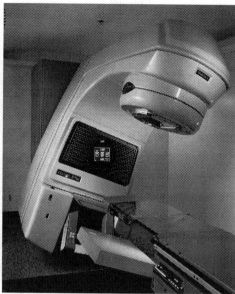

(a) Elekta's Synergy S
(photograph courtesy of Elekta)

(b) Varian's Clinac
(photograph courtesy of Varian Medical Systems)

Fig. 2.6: Classical gantry-based IMRT systems. Both systems feature an MV imager, the Synergy system also has an orthogonally mounted kV imager.

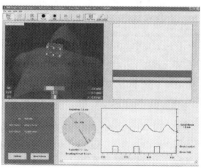
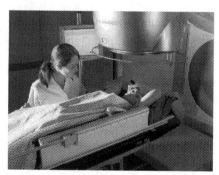

(a) Varian's RPM system
(photograph courtesy of Varian Medical Systems)

(b) Elekta's Active Breathing Coordinator
(photograph courtesy of Elekta)

Fig. 2.7: Commercially available respiratory gating devices

manner, but instead of relying on an external marker box, it uses a combination of stereoscopic X-ray imaging and infrared patient tracking.

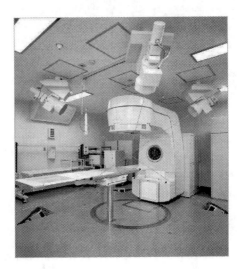

Fig. 2.8: Mitsubishi's RTRT system (photograph courtesy of Hiroki Shirato, Hokkaido University Hospital). Only three of the four X-ray imagers are visible.

A different approach to gating is followed by Elekta's Active Breathing Coordinator™, which requires the patient to actively pause his breathing at pre-defined tidal volumes measured by an aeroplethysmograph. Treatment delivery is subsequently coordinated with this pause (see figure 2.7b) [66]. A similar approach, called Deep Inspiration Breath Hold (DIBH), requires the patient to exhale as much as possible. Gating is then performed at this tidal level [17, 39, 40].

2.3.2 Beam Shaping

The Novalis Tx™ system, manufactured by Varian in cooperation with BrainLAB, see figure 2.9, takes the classical gantry approach one step further by incorporating motion tracking capabilities similar to the CyberKnife system (including stereoscopic X-ray target localisation and respiratory gating). Additionally, it features MV- and kV-imaging as well as MV- and kV-CT. However, this device does not actively compensate for respiratory motion.

Most such systems are based on the principle of Intensity Modulated Radiation Therapy (IMRT) [13, 20]. This method does not use the same beam size and shape throughout the treatment but modifies these parameters for each beam or even during the active time of individual beams. Such modification can be achieved by using

---

[1] Novalis® is a trademark of Brainlab AG in Germany and the US.

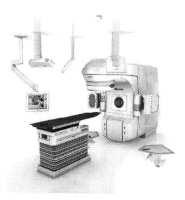

Fig. 2.9: Varian/BrainLAB's Novalis Tx^{TM} system[1] (source: www.brainlab.com)

an MLC [14, 59], a device consisting of multiple metallic leaves made of a high atomic numbered material (usually Wolfram) which can be moved in and out of the beam path to block or attenuate parts of the radiation. An alternative way to shape the beam in IMRT is using physical modulators or compensating filters [28]. Since using such filters is highly cumbersome, their use is not widely spread and they have been described as being an interim technology [20]. Two MLCs and a sketch detailing how the beam shape is modified in a clinical setting are shown in figure 2.10.

This is done to create irradiation fields of varying intensity, which are applied to the patient from different positions. Note that these fields do not necessarily conform to the form of the tumour as seen from the source of radiation (this is also called Beam's Eye View (BEV)). Classically, MLCs were used for CRT and, subsequently, 3DCRT, to spare healthy tissue. They have been incorporated into IMRT planning [23] only recently when computational power became sufficiently high. Using IMRT—as opposed to classical CRT—it has become possible to also treat non-convex tumour shapes, i.e. tumours wrapping around critical structures like the spine or the cochlear nerve. Using gantry-based devices with MLCs, it is also possible to dynamically compensate for organ motion by adapting the MLC shape [24, 30, 31, 36, 38, 67]. Tracking the tumour position can either be done in a similar fashion to the CyberKnife system, i.e. using room-mounted X-ray cameras like it is done in Mitsubishi's RTRT system, or by using an MV imager [55] which is available for most gantry-based systems. On top of this, the manufacturers offer additional kV imaging, mounted orthogonally to the MV treatment tube, to be able to determine the true 3D position of the target. First experiments with this setup were done in [21]. Respiratory motion tracking with combined kV/MV imaging has been shown to be possible [64].

---

[2] m3® is a trademark of Brainlab AG in Germany and the US.

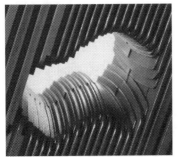

(a) Varian MLC (photograph courtesy of
Varian Medical Systems)

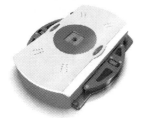

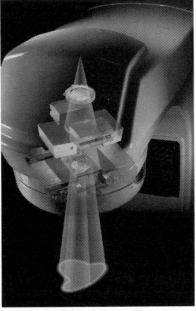

(b) BrainLAB m3® MLC² (source: (c) Beam shaping with Varian's Clinac system
www.brainlab.com)   (photograph courtesy of Varian Medical Systems)

Fig. 2.10: Multi Leaf Collimators and beam shaping

2.4 Tomotherapy

A completely different approach to IMRT uses systems based on CT-scanners. These systems can deliver radiation in a coplanar fashion using an X-ray source. The technology is called tomotherapy, due to its similarity to tomography [27]. *Serial* tomotherapy describes the delivery of multiple fan beams with discrete couch position increments between each axial gantry arc, while in *helical* tomotherapy the gantry and couch motion are synchronised and happen simultaneously (i.e. the source describes a helical trajectory from the patient's point of view) [20, 58]. Tomotherapy devices are manufactured by TomoTherapy, Inc.,[H] (the Hi·Art® system, see figure 2.11a) and Best nomos[I] (the nomosSTAT™ system, see figure 2.11b). The Hi·Art system is a stand-alone machine based on helical tomotherapy and it also incorporates a CT scanner. The nomosSTAT system, on the other hand, is based on serial tomotherapy and is an add-on device to classical gantry-based treatment devices.

To date, respiratory motion compensation using tomotherapy machines is not clinically available. It is a topic under investigation, however, and recent works show that it is feasible to significantly improve plan delivery using motion compensation strategies [25, 26].

---

[3] This work is reproduced and distributed with the permission of Best Medical International, Inc.

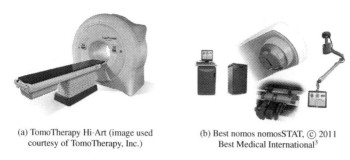

(a) TomoTherapy Hi·Art (image used courtesy of TomoTherapy, Inc.)

(b) Best nomos nomosSTAT, © 2011 Best Medical International[3]

Fig. 2.11: Tomotherapy systems

2.5 The CyberHeart Project

A new application of robotic radiosurgery has been envisioned by Pankratov, Benetti, and Vivian in 2005 [37]. Their patent was subsequently acquired by Thomas J. Fogarty, M.D., who, together with Roderick A. Young, then founded the company CyberHeart, Inc.,[J] dedicated to developing the robotic ablation treatment for cardiac arrhythmia described in this patent. At the moment, the company is investigating the possibility of curing atrial fibrillation by means of radiation.

2.5.1 Medical Background

Atrial fibrillation (ICD-10 code I48), is the single most common manifestation of abnormal heart rhythms. It involves uncoordinated contraction of the muscles of the two upper chambers of the heart. These contractions are triggered by disorganised electrical impulses obscuring the normal excitation generated by the sinoatrial node. These impulses most frequently originate from the atria themselves or from the pulmonary veins. Atrial fibrillation by itself is mostly asymptomatic but results in an increased risk of stroke. Additionally, patients with chronic atrial fibrillation are often subject to cardiac insufficiency. Atrial fibrillation is very common in the general population: about 4.5 million people in the EU suffer from it and 25 % of all people in the EU over 40 years old are expected to develop atrial fibrillation in their life [33].

Atrial fibrillation is, nowadays, usually treated with medication or by synchronised electrical cardioversion. If these methods are not available or have failed, RF ablation is used. The goal of RF ablation is to place lesions on the heart tissue from inside the atria or to remove parts of the muscle bundles around the end of the pulmonary veins. Major disadvantages of RF ablation are frequent side effects, like thromboembolism and stenosis of the pulmonary veins, and the long duration of the intervention. Even so, RF ablation is considered the gold standard in treating atrial fibrillation [1].

2.5.2 Technical Details

Planned as an extension of the CyberKnife system, the CyberHeart project endeavours to cure atrial fibrillation by placing ablation lines around the pulmonary veins to block electrical excitation emanating from these spots. This procedure is to be done on the beating heart using a modified version of the CyberKnife [49]. Feasibility studies and first pre-clinical trials have been done and show promising results [29, 50].

As a consequence, very precise localisation of the pulmonary veins and compensation of both respiratory and pulsatory motion is required. That the detection of the pulmonary veins using live 3D ultrasound actually is possible has been demonstrated [8, 9]. Furthermore, the application of algorithms developed with the goal of human respiratory motion prediction to pulsatory motion will be investigated in section 4.7.

Apart from this novel approach, there also is a limited number of patients who actually suffer from cardiac cancer [56] or tumours which move with pulsation [57]. Treating such lesions will also require detecting and compensating for cardiac motion.

References

[1] ACC/AHA/ESC: ACC/AHA/ESC 2006 guidelines for the management of patients with atrial fibrillation. Circulation **114**(7), e257–354 (2006). DOI 10.1161/CIRCULATIONAHA.106.177292

[2] Adler Jr., J.R.: Interactive image-guided neurosurgery, chap. Image-based frameless stereotactic radiosurgery, pp. 81–89. American Association of Neurological Surgeons (1993)

[3] Adler Jr., J.R.: Clinical neurosurgery, *The Congress of Neurological Surgeons*, vol. 52, chap. Accuray, incorporated: a neurosurgical business case study, pp. 87–96. Lippincott, Williams and Wilkins (2005)

[4] Adler Jr., J.R., Chang, S.D., Murphy, M.J., Doty, J., Geis, P., Hancock, S.L.: The CyberKnife: A frameless robotic system for radiosurgery. Stereotactic and Functional Neurosurgery **69**, 124–128 (1997). DOI 10.1159/000099863

[5] Adler Jr., J.R., Hancock, S.L.: The Neurotron 1000: A system for frameless stereotactic radiosurgery. Perspectives in Neurological Surgery **5**(1), 127–133 (1994)

[6] Adler Jr., J.R., Schweikard, A.: Future health: computers and medicine in the twenty-first century, chap. Bloodless robotic surgery, pp. 123–129. St. Martin's Press, Inc., New York, NY, USA (1995)

[7] Adler Jr., J.R., Schweikard, A., Murphy, M.J., Hancock, S.L.: Image-guided neurosurgery: clinical applications of surgical navigation, chap. Image-guided stereotactic radiosurgery: The CyberKnife, pp. 193–204. Quality Medical Publishing, St. Louis, MO (1998)

[8] Bruder, R., Cai, T., Ernst, F., Schweikard, A.: 3D ultrasound-guided motion compensation for intravascular radiation therapy. In: Proceedings of the 23rd International Conference and Exhibition on Computer Assisted Radiology and Surgery (CARS'09), *International Journal of CARS*, vol. 4, pp. 25–26. CARS, Berlin, Germany (2009). DOI 10.1007/s11548-009-0309-y

[9] Bruder, R., Ernst, F., Schlaefer, A., Schweikard, A.: Real-time tracking of the pulmonary veins in 3D ultrasound of the beating heart. In: 51st Annual Meeting of the AAPM, *Medical Physics*, vol. 36, p. 2804. American Association of Physicists in Medicine, Anaheim, CA, USA (2009). DOI 10.1118/1.3182643. TH-C-304A-07

[10] Chang, S.D., Murphy, M.J., Martin, D.P., Hancock, S.L., Doty, J., Adler Jr., J.R.: Radiosurgery, vol. 3, chap. Image-Guided Robotic Radiosurgery: Clinical and Radiographic Results with the CyberKnife, pp. 23–33. Karger Medical and Scientific Publishers, New York (1999)

[11] D'Souza, W.D., McAvoy, T.J.: An analysis of the treatment couch and control system dynamics for respiration-induced motion compensation. Medical Physics **33**(12), 4701–4709 (2006). DOI 10.1118/1.2372218

[12] D'Souza, W.D., Naqvi, S.A., Yu, C.X.: Real-time intra-fraction-motion tracking using the treatment couch: a feasibility study. Physics in Medicine and Biology **50**(17), 4021–4033 (2005). DOI 10.1088/0031-9155/50/17/007

[13] Galvin, J.M., Ezzell, G., Eisbrauch, A., Yu, C.X., Butler, B., Xiao, Y., Rosen, I., Rosenman, J., Sharpe, M.B., Xing, L., Xia, P., Lomax, T., Low, D.A., Palta, J.: Implementing IMRT in clinical practice: a joint document of the american society for therapeutic radiology and oncology and the american association of physicists in medicine. International Journal of Radiation Oncology, Biology, Physics **58**(5), 1616–1634 (2004). DOI 10.1016/j.ijrobp.2003.12.008

[14] Galvin, J.M., Smith, A.R., Lally, B.: Characterization of a multileaf collimator system. International Journal of Radiation Oncology, Biology, Physics **25**(2), 181–192 (1993)

[15] Guthrie, B.L., Adler Jr., J.R.: Frameless stereotaxy: Computer interactive neurosurgery. Perspectives in Neurological Surgery **2**(1), 1–22 (1991)

[16] Guthrie, B.L., Adler Jr., J.R.: Clinical Neurosurgery, *The Congress of Neurological Surgeons*, vol. 38, chap. Computer-assisted preoperative planning, interactive surgery, and frameless stereotaxy, pp. 112–131. Williams and Wilkins (1992)

[17] Hanley, J., Debois, M.M., Mah, D., Mageras, G.S., Raben, A., Rosenzweig, K., Mychalczak, B., Schwartz, L.H., Gloeggler, P.J., Lutz, W., Ling, C.C., Leibel, S.A., Fuks, Z., Kutcher, G.J.: Deep inspiration breath-hold technique for lung tumors: the potential value of target immobilization and reduced lung density in dose escalation. International Journal of Radiation Oncology, Biology, Physics **45**(3), 603–611 (1999). DOI 10.1016/s0360-3016(99)00154-6

[18] Hirai, E., Tsukuda, K., Kamino, Y., Miura, S., Takayama, K., Aoi, T.: State-of-the-art medical treatment machine MHI-TM2000. Mitsubishi Heavy Industries Technical Review **46**(1), 29–32 (2009)

[19] Hoogeman, M., Prévost, J.B., Nuyttens, J., Pöll, J., Levendag, P., Heijmen, B.: Clinical accuracy of the respiratory tumor tracking system of the CyberKnife: Assessment by analysis of log files. International Journal of Radiation Oncology, Biology, Physics **74**(1), 297–303 (2009). DOI 10.1016/j.ijrobp.2008.12.041

[20] IMRT Collaborative Working Group: Intensity-modulated radiotherapy: current status and issues of interest. International Journal of Radiation Oncology, Biology, Physics **51**(4), 880–914 (2001)

[21] Jaffray, D.A., Drake, D.G., Moreau, M., Martinez, A.A., Wong, J.W.: A radiographic and tomographic imaging system integrated into a medical linear accelerator for localization of bone and soft-tissue targets. International Journal of Radiation Oncology, Biology, Physics **45**(3), 773–789 (1999). DOI 10.1016/s0360-3016(99)00118-2

[22] Kamino, Y., Takayama, K., Kokubo, M., Narita, Y., Hirai, E., Kawada, N., Mizowaki, T., Nagata, Y., Nishidai, T., Hiraoka, M.: Development of a four-dimensional image-guided radiotherapy system with a gimbaled X-ray head. International Journal of Radiation Oncology, Biology, Physics **66**(1), 271–278 (2006). DOI 10.1016/j.ijrobp.2006.04.044

[23] Keall, P.J., Joshi, S., Vedam, S.S., Siebers, J.V., Kini, V.R., Mohan, R.: Four-dimensional radiotherapy planning for DMLC-based respiratory motion tracking. Medical Physics **32**(4), 942–951 (2005). DOI 10.1118/1.1879152

[24] Keall, P.J., Kini, V.R., Vedam, S.S., Mohan, R.: Motion adaptive X-ray therapy: a feasibility study. Physics in Medicine and Biology **46**(1), 1–10 (2001)

[25] Lu, W.: Real-time motion-adaptive delivery (MAD) using binary MLC: II. Rotational beam (tomotherapy) delivery. Physics in Medicine and Biology **53**(22), 6513–6531 (2008)

[26] Lu, W., Chen, M., Ruchala, K.J., Chen, Q., Langen, K.M., Kupelian, P.A., Olivera, G.H.: Real-time motion-adaptive-optimization (MAO) in Tomo-Therapy. Physics in Medicine and Biology **54**(14), 4373–4398 (2009). DOI 10.1088/0031-9155/54/14/003

[27] Mackie, T.R., Holmes, T., Swerdloff, S., Reckwerdt, P., Deasy, J.O., Yang, J., Paliwal, B., Kinsella, T.: Tomotherapy: A new concept for the delivery of dynamic conformal radiotherapy. Medical Physics **20**(6), 1709–1719 (1993). DOI 10.1118/1.596958

[28] Mageras, G.S., Mohan, R., Burman, C., Barest, G.D., Kutcher, G.J.: Compensators for three-dimensional treatment planning. Medical Physics **18**(2), 133–140 (1991). DOI 10.1118/1.596699

[29] Maguire, P., Sharma, A., Fogarty, T., Sumanaweera, T., Jack, A.: Non-invasive radiosurgical ablation of the myocardium: Pre clinical electrophysiology and histology. In: Boston Atrial Fibrillation Symposium (2008)

[30] McClelland, J.R., Webb, S., McQuaid, D., Binnie, D.M., Hawkes, D.J.: Tracking 'differential organ motion' with a 'breathing' multileaf collimator: magnitude of problem assessed using 4D CT data and a motion-compensation strategy. Physics in Medicine and Biology **52**(16), 4805–4826 (2007). DOI 10.1088/0031-9155/52/16/007

[31] McQuaid, D., Webb, S.: IMRT delivery to a moving target by dynamic MLC tracking: delivery for targets moving in two dimensions in the beam's eye view. Physics in Medicine and Biology **51**(19), 4819–4839 (2006). DOI 10.1088/0031-9155/51/19/007

[32] Mehta, M.P., Noyes, W.R., Mackie, T.R.: Linear accelerator configurations for radiosurgery. Seminars in Radiation Oncology **5**(3), 203–212 (1995). DOI 10.1016/s1053-4296(05)80018-9. Stereotactic Radiosurgery

[33] Mewis, C., Neuberger, H.R., Böhm, M.: Vorhofflimmern. Deutsche Medizinische Wochenschrift **131**(50), 2843–2854 (2006). DOI 10.1055/s-2006-957212

[34] Mitsubishi Heavy Industries, Ltd.: MHI's first radiotherapy machine for overseas to begin treatment at Brussels University Hospital (UZ Brussel). Press release (2009). URL http://www.mhi.co.jp/en/news/story/0912031325.html. MHI News No. 1325

[35] Muacevic, A., Staehler, M., Drexler, C., Wowra, B., Reiser, M., Tonn, J.C.: Technical description, phantom accuracy, and clinical feasibility for fiducial-free frameless real-time image-guided spinal radiosurgery. Journal of Neurosurgery **5**(4), 303–312 (2006). DOI 10.3171/spi.2006.5.4.303. PMID: 17048766

[36] Neicu, T., Shirato, H., Seppenwoolde, Y., Jiang, S.B.: Synchronized moving aperture radiation therapy (SMART): average tumour trajectory for lung patients. Physics in Medicine and Biology **48**(5), 587–598 (2003). DOI 10.1088/0031-9155/48/5/303

[37] Pankratov, M., Benetti, F., Vivian, J.: Method for non-invasive heart treatment (2005). U.S. patent 6,889,695

[38] Papież, L.: DMLC leaf-pair optimal control of IMRT delivery for a moving rigid target. Medical Physics **31**(10), 2742–2754 (2004). DOI 10.1118/1.1779358

[39] Rosenzweig, K.E., Hanley, J., Mah, D., Mageras, G.S., Hunt, M., Toner, S., Burman, C., Ling, C.C., Mychalczak, B., Fuks, Z., Leibel, S.A.: The deep inspiration breath-hold technique in the treatment of inoperable non-small-cell lung cancer. International Journal of Radiation Oncology, Biology, Physics **48**(1), 81–87 (2000). DOI 10.1016/s0360-3016(00)00583-6

[40] Rosenzweig, K.E., Hanley, J., Mychalczak, B., Fuks, Z., Mageras, G.S., Yorke, E., Ling, C.C., Burman, C., Ginsberg, R.J., Kris, M.G., Leibel, S.A.: Phase i dose escalation study using the deep inspiration breath hold technique to safely increase dose to 81 gy in the treatment of inoperable non-small cell lung cancer. International Journal of Radiation Oncology, Biology, Physics **48**(3, supp. 1), 233–233 (2000). DOI 10.1016/S0360-3016(00)80260-6

[41] Schweikard, A., Adler Jr., J.R., Latombe, J.C.: Motion planning in stereotaxic radiosurgery. IEEE Transactions on Robotics and Automation **9**(6), 764–774 (1993). DOI 10.1109/70.265920

[42] Schweikard, A., Bodduluri, M., Adler Jr., J.R.: Planning for camera-guided robotic radiosurgery. IEEE Transactions on Robotics and Automation **14**(6), 951–962 (1998). DOI 10.1109/70.736778

[43] Schweikard, A., Glosser, G., Bodduluri, M., Murphy, M.J., Adler Jr., J.R.: Robotic Motion Compensation for Respiratory Movement during Radiosurgery. Journal of Computer-Aided Surgery **5**(4), 263–277 (2000). DOI 10.3109/10929080009148894

[44] Schweikard, A., Shiomi, H., Adler Jr., J.R.: Respiration tracking in radiosurgery. Medical Physics **31**(10), 2738–2741 (2004). DOI 10.1118/1.1774132

[45] Schweikard, A., Shiomi, H., Adler Jr., J.R.: Respiration tracking in radiosurgery without fiducials. International Journal of Medical Robotics and Computer Assisted Surgery **1**(2), 19–27 (2005). DOI 10.1002/rcs.38

[46] Schweikard, A., Shiomi, H., Uchida, M., Adler Jr., J.R.: Extracranial Stereotactic Radiotherapy and Radiosurgery, chap. Whole-Body Radiosurgery with the Cyberknife, pp. 71–87. Taylor and Francis, New York (2005)

[47] Schweikard, A., Tombropoulos, R., Kavraki, L., Adler Jr., J.R., Latombe, J.C.: Treatment planning for a radiosurgical system with general kinematics. In: IEEE International Conference on Robotics and Automation (ICRA 1994), pp. 1720–1727 (1994). DOI 10.1109/robot.1994.351344

[48] Seppenwoolde, Y., Berbeco, R.I., Nishioka, S., Shirato, H., Heijmen, B.: Accuracy of tumor motion compensation algorithm from a robotic respiratory tracking system: A simulation study. Medical Physics **34**(7), 2774–2784 (2007). DOI 10.1118/1.2739811

[49] Sharma, A., Maguire, P., Sumanaweera, T., Wong, D., Marshall, R., Fajardo, L., Fogarty, T.: Non-invasive ablation of the left superior pulmonary vein-left atrial junction using stereotactic focussed radiation. Circulation **116**, II 489 (2007)

[50] Sharma, A., Maguire, P., Wong, D., Sumanaweera, T., Steele, J., Peterson, P., Fajardo, L., Takeda, P., Fogarty, T.: New non-invasive therapy for cardiac arrhythmias using stereotactic radiosurgery: Initial feasibility testing. In: 2007 Heart Rhythm Symposium, *Heart Rhythm*, vol. 4, p. S68 (2007)

[51] Shirato, H., Oita, M., Fujita, K., Watanabe, Y., Miyasaka, K.: Feasibility of synchronization of real-time tumor-tracking radiotherapy and intensity-modulated radiotherapy from viewpoint of excessive dose from fluoroscopy. International Journal of Radiation Oncology, Biology, Physics **60**(1), 335 – 341 (2004). DOI 10.1016/j.ijrobp.2004.04.028

[52] Shirato, H., Shimizu, S., Kitamura, K., Nishioka, T., Kagei, K., Hashimoto, S., Aoyama, H., Kunieda, T., Shinohara, N., Dosaka-Akita, H., Miyasaka, K.: Four-dimensional treatment planning and fluoroscopic real-time tumor tracking radiotherapy for moving tumor. International Journal of Radiation Oncology, Biology, Physics **48**(2), 435–442 (2000). DOI 10.1016/s0360-3016(00)00625-8

[53] Shirato, H., Shimizu, S., Kunieda, T., Kitamura, K., van Herk, M., Kagei, K., Nishioka, T., Hashimoto, S., Fujita, K., Aoyama, H., Tsuchiya, K., Kudo, K., Miyasaka, K.: Physical aspects of a real-time tumor-tracking system for gated radiotherapy. International Journal of Radiation Oncology, Biology, Physics **48**(4), 1187 – 1195 (2000). DOI 10.1016/s0360-3016(00)00748-3

[54] Shirato, H., Shimizu, S., Shimizu, T., Nishioka, T., Miyasaka, K.: Real-time tumour-tracking radiotherapy. The Lancet **353**(9161), 1331 – 1332 (1999). DOI 10.1016/s0140-6736(99)00700-x

[55] Simpson, R.G., Chen, C.T., Grubbs, E.A., Swindell, W.: A 4-MV CT scanner for radiation therapy: The prototype system. Medical Physics **9**(4), 574–579 (1982). DOI 10.1118/1.595102

[56] Smith, R.: World's first heart surgery using radiation. telegraph.co.uk (02.11.2009). URL http://www.telegraph.co.uk/journalists/rebecca-smith/6469279/Worlds-first-heart-surgery-using-radiation.html

[57] Soltys, S.G., Kalani, M.Y.S., Cheshier, S.H., Szabo, K.A., Lo, A., Chang, S.D.: Stereotactic radiosurgery for a cardiac sarcoma: A case report. Technology in Cancer Research and Treatment **7**(5), 363–367 (2008)

[58] Sterzing, F., Schubert, K., Sroka-Perez, G., Kalz, J., Debus, J., Herfarth, K.: Helical tomotherapy. Strahlentherapie und Onkologie **184**(1), 8–14 (2008). DOI 10.1007/s00066-008-1778-6

[59] Takahashi, S.: Conformation radiotherapy: rotation techniques as applied to radiography and radiotherapy of cancer. Acta radiologica: diagnosis **supp. 242**, 1–142 (1965)

[60] Takayama, K., Mizowaki, T., Kokubo, M., Kawada, N., Nakayama, H., Narita, Y., Nagano, K., Kamino, Y., Hiraoka, M.: Initial validations for pursuing irradiation using a gimbals tracking system. Radiotherapy and Oncology **93**(1), 45–49 (2009). DOI 10.1016/j.radonc.2009.07.011

[61] Universitair Ziekenhuis Brussel: UZ Brussel inaugurates Vero high precision radiation therapy system. Press release (2009). URL http://www.uzbrussel.be/u/view/en/3000848-UZ+Brussel+inaugurates+Vero+High+Precision+Radiation+Therapy+System.html

[62] Urschel Jr., H.C., Kresl, J.J., Luketich, J.D., Papież, L., Timmerman, R.D. (eds.): Robotic Radiosurgery. Treating Tumors that Move with Respiration, 1st edn. Springer, Berlin (2007). DOI 10.1007/978-3-540-69886-9

[63] VHL Family Alliance: Robot does brain surgery. VHL Family Forum **2**(3), 1–2 (1994). URL http://www.vhl.org/newsletter/vhl1994/94caster.php

[64] Wiersma, R.D., Mao, W., Xing, L.: Combined kV and MV imaging for real-time tracking of implanted fiducial markers. Medical Physics **35**(4), 1191–1198 (2008). DOI 10.1118/1.2842072

[65] Wilbert, J., Meyer, J., Baier, K., Guckenberger, M., Herrmann, C., Hess, R., Janka, C., Ma, L., Mersebach, T., Richter, A., Roth, M., Schilling, K., Flentje, M.: Tumor tracking and motion compensation with an adaptive tumor tracking system (ATTS): system description and prototype testing. Medical Physics **35**(9), 3911–3921 (2008). DOI 10.1118/1.2964090

[66] Wong, J.W., Sharpe, M.B., Jaffray, D.A., Kini, V.R., Robertson, J.M., Stromberg, J.S., Martinez, A.A.: The use of active breathing control (ABC) to reduce margin for breathing motion. International Journal of Radiation Oncology,

Biology, Physics **44**(4), 911–919 (1999). DOI 10.1016/s0360-3016(99)00056-5

[67] Xu, J., Papanikolaou, N., Shi, C., Jiang, S.B.: Synchronized moving aperture radiation therapy (SMART): superimposing tumor motion on IMRT MLC leaf sequences under realistic delivery conditions. Physics in Medicine and Biology **54**(16), 4993–5007 (2009). DOI 10.1088/0031-9155/54/16/010

Chapter 3
Signal Processing[1]

Actively compensating for respiratory and pulsatory motion—as outlined in section 2.5—requires real time tracking of marker positions on the patient's chest and subsequent prediction (see chapter 4) and correlation (see chapter 5). It is clear that we deal with some kind of control process: the robot is moved in real time according to processed sensory input from the tracking system. To quantify the accuracy of the individual processing steps, new evaluation metrics are introduced (section 3.2), a new method to reduce measurement noise will be discussed (section 3.3, published in [7, 10]), the noise level of different tracking systems will be evaluated (section 3.4) and motion artefacts inherent to active optical cameras will be analysed (section 3.5, published in [8]).

3.1 Determining the Latency

Since we do not have access to a CyberKnife, we have tried to identify sources of systematic latency in greater detail using similar hardware in our laboratory.

3.1.1 Experiment: Latency of Optical Tracking Devices

One source of latency in robotic radiosurgery is the time between motion of the patient's chest (and the optical markers on the chest) and the moment when the motion is detected in the control software. In our laboratory, we have measured this delay. We used the accuTrack 250 system[(K)] (shown in figure B.2 of appendix B), and a custom-built marker of one Light Emitting Diode (LED). We then attached a two-channel oscilloscope to the wires connecting the LED to the tracking system and to the output of a relay switchable via an RS-232 port (connected to the acquisition

---

[1] Parts of this chapter have been published in [7, 8, 10, 20]

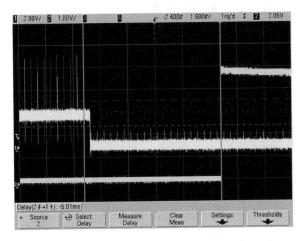

Fig. 3.1: Determination of the latency of the Atracsys accuTrack 250 system, operating at 4.1 kHz. Yellow (spiky): voltage provided to the LED, green: output of the relay. It was triggered as soon as the LED became invisible to the software. Vertical lines: latency measured between the last LED pulse and the trigger signal's shoulder

PC using high-speed USB). Using this setup, we can clearly see the voltage peaks of the LED (figure 3.1, left) and the flat signal of the relay's output (figure 3.1, left). To determine the latency, a computer programme running on ubuntu 8.04 with real time kernel continuously polled the tracking system for the position of the LED. Then the LED was switched off (drop in baseline of the spiky curve in figure 3.1) and the programme triggered the relay as soon as the LED was reported as invisible (jump in the flat curve in figure 3.1). With this setup, the maximal latency of the tracking system—when operating at 4.1 kHz—was determined as approximately 5 ms. This is the time between the last LED peak and the shoulder of the relay's output (marked with vertical lines in figure 3.1). Clearly, the accuracy of the setup is limited by several factors:

- Switching off the LED does not necessarily occur directly after the last pulse. This causes an additional delay of up to $1/f$ where f is the frame rate the system operates at. The accuTrack can operate between 331.04 and 4,111.84 Hz, resulting in a maximal additional delay of up to 3.02 ms (331.04 Hz) and 0.24 ms (4,111.84 Hz).
- The reaction time of the relay is unknown but assumed to be very small, i.e. much smaller than 1 ms.
- The time which passes between the programme sending the trigger signal (i.e. writing to /dev/ttyACM0 in our case) via the RS-232 connection and the arrival of the signal at the relay is unknown.

Altogether, we can say that the total latency of the accuTrack system is below 10 ms and over 4.5 ms.

3.1.2 Experiment: Latency of the Robotic Setup

The second source of latency in robotic radiosurgery is the delay between sending a motion command to the robot controller and the robot reaching the new position. Since we do not have access to a CyberKnife system, we used a setup with an Adept Viper s850$^{(L)}$ robot, shown in figure B.13 of appendix B.

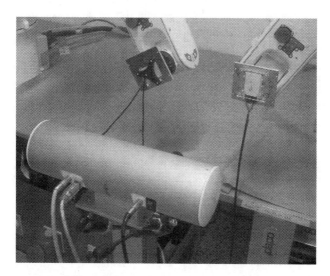

Fig. 3.2: Setup of the robotic latency test

The control loop used to determine the combined latency of communication with the robot, robot controller computation time, and robot motion consists of several parts: we used two identical robots placed next to each other. To each robot, we attached a tracking LED connected to the accuTrack system. Both robots were calibrated to the tracking camera. The LEDs' positions were recorded using our tracking framework [15]. The second (right) robot was controlled using our lab's robot control software (rob6server, a common robot controlling framework designed for adept Viper s850, KUKA KR3 and KR16, Kawasaki FS03N [20]). The first robot was then moved using its Manual Control Pendant (MCP). The second robot was controlled by a programme to follow the motion of the first robot as detected by the tracking system. The procedure is outlined below.

- First robot moves
- Motion detected by tracking camera
- Position $\mathbf{P}_1 = (x_1, y_1, z_1)$ of Robot 1 is computed using calibration information
- Target position $\mathbf{P}_2$ of the second robot is computed as $\mathbf{P}_2 = (-x_1, y_1, z_1)$
- The second robot is moved to $\mathbf{P}_2$

Both LEDs' positions were recorded independently and the time shift between the motion trajectories of the two LEDs was evaluated as the combined latency. Figure 3.2 shows the setup of this test.

The results of this experiment can be seen in figure 3.3. The time delay between these two curves was found to be approximately 100 ms. Further experiments, using simple ping-pong commands to both the tracking and robot servers as well as to the robot from the robot server, helped in determining the latency caused by network communication (both 0.25 ms to the robot and the tracking server, 3.2 ms to the robot controller). Timing commands on a client programme running on ubuntu 8.04 with a real time kernel showed the individual computation times (0.1 ms in the client programme, 0.25 ms in the tracking server and 2.5 ms in the robot server). An overview of all latencies determined is given in figure 3.4.

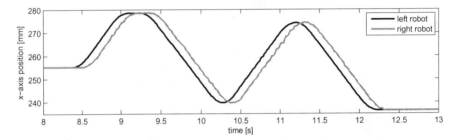

Fig. 3.3: Results of the latency measurements

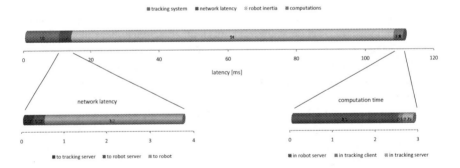

Fig. 3.4: Combined latency of the complete simulation setup. The top graph shows the individual parts of the system latency of 110 ms: network communication, marker acquisition time, robot inertia and computation time. The bottom graphs explain the individual components of the network latency and the different computations involved.

3.2 Evaluation Measures

In all applications described in this work, we need to compare the output of different algorithms (like prediction or correlation) to some kind of ground truth. Similarly, when we analyse the noise characteristics of different tracking systems, which will be done in section 3.4, we want to see how the characteristics of the processed signals have changed with respect to the original signals. To this end, several evaluation measures are introduced here. We will focus on the following main signal characteristics:

1. *Error level*: the single most important characteristic of prediction and correlation is the accuracy of the algorithms' output. We wish to measure this accuracy in terms of *average accuracy* with penalisation of very large errors, in terms of *maximal error* and *confidence intervals* and in terms of *randomness* of the error.
2. *Signal smoothness and stability*: this characteristic is especially important for clinical applicability: the ultimate goal is that a robotic manipulator or the leaves of an MLC can follow the computed motion trajectory. This is only possible if the trajectory is well-behaved, i.e., all motion is within the limits of the machine as defined by the manufacturer. We will measure signal smoothness and stability by means of the *jitter*.
3. *Speed*: also of interest is the runtime needed when applications like prediction, correlation and smoothing come into the signal processing chain. The devices have to operate in real-time and thus it is crucial not to increase the system's latency by slow algorithms.

We will now focus on these different measures.

3.2.1 Measuring the error level[2]

To evaluate the error level of noisy signals or of predicted signals, we introduce a measure commonly used in signal processing: the Root Mean Square (RMS) value, which is defined according to definition 1.

Definition 1 (Root Mean Square). Let s_i, $i = 1, \dots, N$, be an equidistantly sampled signal. The quantity

$$\mathrm{RMS}(s) = \sqrt{\frac{1}{N} \sum_{i=1}^{N} \|s_i\|^2}$$

will be called the *root mean square* or *RMS* of s.

It is important to note that, in contrast to the mean value or mean absolute value, the RMS error penalises larger errors of s_i due to squaring.

---

[2] Parts of this section have been published in [9].

When we look at the quality of predicted signals, a measure derived from RMS is useful, the so-called relative RMS.

Definition 2 (Relative RMS). Let y be the signal to predict, let δ be the prediction horizon and let r be a reference signal. Then the relative RMS is defined as:

$$\text{RMS}_{\text{rel}}(y, r, \delta) = \frac{\text{RMS}(\text{pred}(y, \delta) - r)}{\text{RMS}(D(y, \delta) - r)}$$

Note that $D(y, \delta)$ denotes the signal y delayed by δ samples and $\text{pred}(y, \delta)$ denotes the signal y predicted by δ samples.

In fact, the relative RMS tells us the amount of improvement we can achieve by using a prediction algorithm: if the relative RMS is equal to 0.75 (i.e., 75 %), say, we can deduce that the algorithm employed was capable to reduce the error from the system's latency by 25 % when compared to doing no prediction.

Unfortunately, we know from previous work [6, 11] that the RMS value alone is insufficient for describing the errors of a predicted signal or the output of correlation models. The major problem is that most such algorithms result in very good prediction or correlation along the flanks of the respiratory motion trace (i.e., during inhalation and exhalation) while failing to some extent at those points where the motion changes (like end-of-inhalation or end-of-exhalation). Using RMS, we cannot discern between errors that occur more or less randomly throughout the respiratory cycle and errors which have some kind of periodicity. Additionally, we have no information about the distribution of the error since very different error distributions may result in similar RMS values.

As an example, many plans in radiation therapy feature very steep gradients, either to protect OARs or to increase local tumour control. In this setting, the magnitude and distribution of errors is not irrelevant and do not necessarily average out over time. Assume a situation where an OAR is close to a steep gradient, let's say 0.6 mm away. Then an RMS error of 0.5 mm will sound acceptable. Now consider the following signals:

$$s_1(t) = \begin{cases} 0.3\,\text{mm} & \text{for } t < 0.6 \\ 0.7\,\text{mm} & \text{for } t \geq 0.6 \end{cases}$$

$$s_2(t) = 0.5\,\text{mm for all } t$$

Here, t ranges from 0 to 1 and the signals should be understood as motion of the gradient towards the OAR.

Both signals have an RMS of 0.5 mm, but with s_1 the OAR will be hit by too much dose in 40 % of the cases. This explains why additional measures capturing more of the error signal's properties have to be introduced. One of them is the notion of confidence intervals (not to be confounded with confidence intervals as used in statistics), defined below.

Definition 3 (Confidence intervals). Let s_i, $i = 1, \ldots, N$, be an equidistantly sampled signal and let $0 < d \leq 1$. Then we define the *d-confidence interval* (or *CI-d*) of *s* as

$$\mathrm{CI}(d,s) = \underset{\varepsilon \geq 0}{\mathrm{argmin}} \left(\frac{\#\{1 \leq i \leq N : |s_i| \leq \varepsilon\}}{N} \geq d \right).$$

Here, the operator $\#\{\dots\}$ denotes the number of elements in a set.

As an example, the value $\mathrm{CI}(0.5, s)$ is the smallest number ε so $|s_i| \leq \varepsilon$ for at least 50 % of the indices $i = 1,\dots,N$. Consequently, when we look at the output of a prediction algorithm, we can thus determine the error that is not exceeded in 90 % of the cases, say, by computing $\mathrm{CI}(0.9, \mathrm{pred}\,(y, \delta) - y)$.

With this measure we now have the means of more accurately classifying the distribution of errors of predicted or correlated output. One problem, however, remains: as mentioned before, it is of clinical relevance to determine whether errors are purely random or have some kind of periodicity or regularity. If, as an example, a certain prediction algorithm constantly underestimates the organ position at peak inhalation, the radiosurgery system would systematically over- and underdose parts of the tumour and/or healthy tissue. This is crucial, since there is a trend towards hypofractionated therapy [16, 18] in which these treatment errors cannot average out over time, since the patient comes to treatment only once or, at most, a couple of times.

One thing that immediately comes to mind when trying to quantify the periodicity of a signal is to look at the signal's spectrum. Using a Discrete Fourier Transform (DFT), this spectrum can be computed quite easily. We would now like to use the spectrum to determine whether an error signal has periodic components, and if so, how strong they are. Let us assume that we have computed the power spectrum P of a signal y. If we now only look at those frequencies with "high" energies, i.e., $P > \tau$ for some τ, and compute the relation of these frequencies' energy and the spectrum's total energy, we can estimate the contribution of these frequencies to the error. The first idea of defining an error measure on a signal's spectrum is now given in definition 4.

Definition 4 (Error measure on the spectrum, I). Let s_i, $i = 1,\dots,N$, be an equidistantly sampled signal and let f_j and P_j, $j = 1,\dots,N/2+1 =: M$, be the signal's spectrum computed by DFT, i.e., f are the determined frequencies and P the corresponding spectral powers. We can now define the ε-*Frequency Content* (or FC^I-ε) of *s* as

$$FC^I(s, \varepsilon) = \frac{\sum_{j \in \Omega} P_j}{\sum_{j=1}^{M} P_j},$$

where

$$\Omega = \left\{ 1 \leq j \leq M : P_j \geq \min_j P_j + (1 - \varepsilon) \left(\max_j P_j - \min_j P_j \right) \right\}.$$

To explain Ω, let ε be 0.1. Then Ω contains the indices of the frequencies with "high" energy, i.e., whose energy is larger than 90 % of the highest energy seen in the spectrum.

This measure should enable us to discern between purely random signals and signals with high regularity. Since the spectrum of Gaussian white noise is independently Gaussian in both real and imaginary components, its power spectrum follows a Rayleigh distribution. If we now use moderate values for ε, like 0.1 or 0.3, say, the frequency content of white Gaussian noise is going to be very small. This is illustrated in figure 3.5.

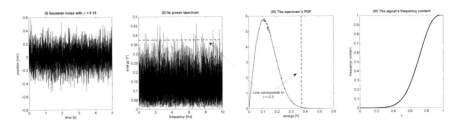

Fig. 3.5: This figure shows Gaussian noise with $\sigma = 0.15$ (I), its power spectrum (II), the power spectrum's PDF (III), and the frequency content of the signal as a function of ε (IV). The PDF follows a Rayleigh distribution and frequency content is, in fact, a variation of the spectrum's CDF.

Unfortunately, using this definition, we can run into difficulties when using real breathing motion traces: the problem is that we don't have properly periodic signals but that the period lengths change unpredictably. This can be circumvented by not regarding the signals as functions of time but of phase and by resampling the signals so each period is represented by an equal number of samples, i.e., that the phase is equidistantly sampled. Consequently, the DFT is now computed on the resampled signal.

Clearly, this approach will result in an "averaged" spectrum, i.e., the frequencies computed are those of an average respiratory cycle.

Definition 5 (Error measure on the spectrum, II). Let s and N be as in definition 4. Now let s be divided into K disjoint periods S_k, $k = 1, \ldots, K$, with n_k samples each, i.e. $S_k = \left(S_{k,1}, \ldots, S_{k,n_k}\right)^{\mathrm{T}}$, $N = \sum_{k=1}^{K} n_k$ and $s = \left(S_1^{\mathrm{T}}, S_2^{\mathrm{T}}, \ldots, S_K^{\mathrm{T}}\right)^{\mathrm{T}}$. Let $\bar{n} = \lceil N/K \rceil$ be the average length of a period. Now let $\tilde{S}_k$ be an equidistantly resampled version of S_k such that $\tilde{S}_k$ has exactly $\bar{n}$ samples and let $\tilde{s} = \left(\tilde{S}_1^{\mathrm{T}}, \tilde{S}_2^{\mathrm{T}}, \ldots, \tilde{S}_K^{\mathrm{T}}\right)^{\mathrm{T}}$. Then

$$\mathrm{FC}^{\mathrm{II}}\left(s, \varepsilon\right) = \frac{\sum_{j \in \Omega} \tilde{P}_j}{\sum_{j=1}^{M} \tilde{P}_j},$$

where $\tilde{P}$ is the power spectrum of the DFT of $\tilde{s}$ and Ω is defined as in definition 4 using $\tilde{P}$ instead of P.

Using this modified definition, accounting for changing respiratory frequencies has become possible.

Another problem is that the spectrum can be badly contaminated by noise. To this end, we compute a smoothed version of the spectrum according to the following definition.

Definition 6 (Decimating the Spectrum). Let P_j, $j = 1, \ldots, M$ be the power spectrum of a signal y and let $R \in \mathbb{N}$. Then we can define the R-decimated spectrum P^{decim} as

$$P_j^{\mathrm{decim}} = \frac{1}{R} \sum_{n=1}^{R} P_{R(j-1)+n}, \quad j = 1, \ldots, \lfloor M/R \rfloor - 1,$$

i.e., P^{decim} is the running average of P computed over R samples.

One thing that might still occlude some information is the fact that the ratio between time spent at inhalation and time spent at exhalation might also change. Since we wish to treat errors during inspiration and expiration equally, this should also be compensated for in our measure.

Definition 7 (Error measure on the spectrum, III). Let s, N, K, and S_k be as in definition 5. Furthermore, divide each period S_k into disjoint inhalation and exhalation parts $S_k^\uparrow$ and $S_k^\downarrow$ with lengths $n_k^\uparrow$ and $n_k^\downarrow$, respectively. Let $\bar{n}^\uparrow$ be the average length of the inhalation parts and let $\bar{n}^\downarrow$ be the average length of the exhalation parts. Now let $\tilde{S}_k^\uparrow$ and $\tilde{S}_k^\downarrow$ be resampled versions of $S_k^\uparrow$ and $S_k^\downarrow$ having $\bar{n}^\uparrow$ and $\bar{n}^\downarrow$ samples, respectively. Now let $\tilde{s}^{\updownarrow} = \left(\tilde{S}_1^{\uparrow\,\mathrm{T}}, \tilde{S}_1^{\downarrow\,\mathrm{T}}, \tilde{S}_2^{\uparrow\,\mathrm{T}}, \tilde{S}_2^{\downarrow\,\mathrm{T}}, \ldots, \tilde{S}_K^{\uparrow\,\mathrm{T}}, \tilde{S}_K^{\downarrow\,\mathrm{T}} \right)^{\mathrm{T}}$. Then the DFT of $\tilde{s}^{\updownarrow}$ is computed, i.e., $\tilde{P}^{\updownarrow}$ and $\tilde{f}^{\updownarrow}$ are determined. Let $\tilde{P}^{\updownarrow,\mathrm{decim}}$ be an R-decimated version of $\tilde{P}^{\updownarrow}$.

Then the final version of the frequency content measure is defined as

$$\mathrm{FC}^{\mathrm{III}}(s, \varepsilon) = \frac{\sum_{j \in \Omega} \tilde{P}_j^{\updownarrow,\mathrm{decim}}}{\sum_{j=1}^{M} \tilde{P}_j^{\updownarrow,\mathrm{decim}}},$$

where Ω is defined as in definition 4 using $\tilde{P}^{\updownarrow,\mathrm{decim}}$ instead of P.

Note that in the above definition, R can—in theory—be selected arbitrarily. Our experiments, however, have shown that it is reasonable to decimate the spectrum such that a frequency resolution of 0.05 Hz is not under-run. This can be achieved by selecting

$$R = \left\lfloor \frac{0.05\mathrm{Hz}}{\Delta f} \right\rfloor,$$

where Δf is the spectral resolution of the signal $\tilde{P}^{\updownarrow}$.

It should be noted that the parameter ε in the definitions of FC^{I}, $\mathrm{FC}^{\mathrm{II}}$, and $\mathrm{FC}^{\mathrm{III}}$ can be selected by the user depending on how much frequency-dependence in the error is acceptable.

We will now show that it is indeed possible to find signals which are very different yet have similiar or even the same values for one or more of the introduced measures.

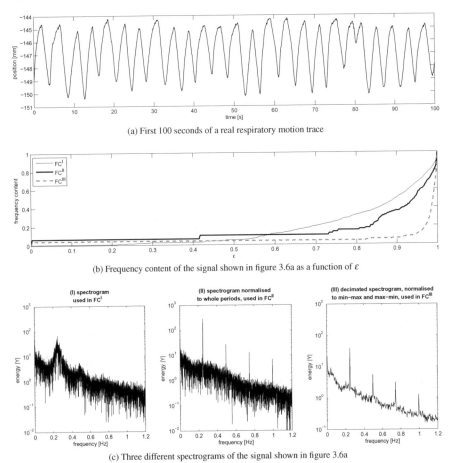

(a) First 100 seconds of a real respiratory motion trace

(b) Frequency content of the signal shown in figure 3.6a as a function of ε

(c) Three different spectrograms of the signal shown in figure 3.6a

Fig. 3.6: First 100 seconds of a real respiratory motion trace (figure 3.6a), its frequency content (figure 3.6b) as a function of ε, and the three different spetrograms (figure 3.6c) used to compute FC^I, FC^{II}, and FC^{III}.

Example 1. Consider a real respiratory signal, x. This signal has been recorded during a CyberKnife treatment session. It is sampled at 26 Hz and has a length of about 45 minutes. Figure 3.6a shows the first 100 seconds of this signal. Now, for $\varepsilon = 0, \ldots, 1$, the values of FC^I-ε, FC^{II}-ε and FC^{III}-ε were computed. They are shown in figure 3.6b. To demonstrate the significance of the normalisation and decimation methods used for the FC-measures, consider figure 3.6c: it shows three spectrograms computed with different normalisation and decimation settings. Part (I) is the original spectrum. Part (II) shows the signal after resampling to complete periods (i.e., as described in definition 5). Part (III) shows the signal after resampling to inspiration and expiration (i.e., as described in definition 7) with decimation to 0.05 Hz. Note that the power is plotted logarithmically.

It is immediately clear that part (I) of figure 3.6c does not reveal much about the signal. Already in part (II) we can see more of the signal's periodicity and part (III) clearly reveals the average frequency and its harmonics.

Example 2. Let x be a simulated respiratory signal, 1,000 seconds long and sampled at 1 kHz. Inspiration is modelled as $2\sin^8(2\pi \cdot 0.125 \cdot t)$ and expiration is modelled as $2\sin^4(2\pi \cdot 0.125 \cdot t)$. More on modelling respiratory signals can be found in appendix D. Furthermore, let v be Gaussian white noise with $\sigma = 0.15$. We can now define four signals such that the differences between x and these signals all have the same RMS:

- $x + v$
- $w \cdot x$, $w = 0.8453$
- $D(x, 111)$, the signal x delayed by 111 samples
- x^A, a signal where each period X_k of x is scaled with a different random factor $A_k \in [0.75, 1.25]$

The following measures have been computed for these signals:
    RMS, CI-0.50, CI-0.75, CI-0.95, FC^{III}-0.10, FC^{III}-0.30
The results are shown in table 3.1. Additionally, figure 3.7 shows the histograms of the differences between the simulated signal x and the four other signals. It immediately becomes clear that, even though the signals have the same RMS error, some of the other characteristics differ strongly and the histograms are clearly distinct. The CI-0.50 values show that the signals x^A and $w \cdot x$ stay very close to the original signal x for most of the samples while the other two signals have already drifted away substantially. When looking at the large CIs, however, we can see that this difference diminishes and, for CI-0.95, even reverses: x^A has both the largest and smallest errors. This is confirmed by looking at its histogram. The clearest difference between the signals can be seen in the FC^{III}-0.10 values: since $x - w \cdot x$ and $x - D(x, 111)$ are both perfectly periodic ($x - w \cdot x$ is made up from one frequency and some weak harmonics, $x - D(x, 111)$ consists of the same frequency plus multiple very strong harmonics), their FC^{III}-0.10 values are very large. On the other hand, $x - (x + v)$ has no periodicity and hence a very low FC^{III}-0.10. Similar conclusions can be drawn from the values of FC^{III}-0.30.

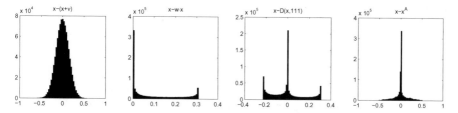

Fig. 3.7: Histograms of the four error signals from example 2

Table 3.1: Error measures for the signals defined in example 2

signal	RMS	CI-0.50	CI-0.75	CI-0.95	FC^{III}-0.10	FC^{III}-0.30
$x-(x+v)$	0.1500	0.1011	0.1726	0.2940	0.0006	0.0006
$x-w\cdot x$	0.1500	0.0452	0.2004	0.3043	0.6687	0.6687
$x-D(x,111)$	0.1500	0.0936	0.2028	0.2952	0.4520	0.7885
$x-x^{\Lambda}$	0.1500	0.0252	0.1411	0.3647	0.0874	0.2322

3.2.2 Signal smoothness and stability

Since the CyberKnife is based on the medical version of a standard industrial robot (KUKA KR 240, see www.kuka.de), the control software has to take into account the manufacturer's specifications. The robot is controlled via a real time TCP/IP link and KUKA's Ethernet RSI XML protocol. Using this protocol, the robot must be provided with a new position every 12 ms, this is the system's internal clock rate [14]. With this in mind, we define a measure used to quantify the *noisiness* of signals.

Definition 8 (Jitter). Let s_i, $i = 1, \ldots, N$, be an equidistantly sampled signal. The quantity

$$\mathfrak{J}(s) = \frac{1}{(N-2)\Delta t} \sum_{i=1}^{N-1} \|s_i - s_{i+1}\|$$

will be called the *jitter of s*. Here, Δt is the temporal spacing between two samples of the signal.

In fact, the jitter is the average distance a robot following a signal would have to move per second. It thus is a measure to describe the amount of change that we expect to occur, i.e. an indication as to how far the signal's first derivative is from being constant. Using the jitter and the robot's clock rate, we can thus determine whether the average distance the robot would have to move in each cycle is acceptable.
In a similar fashion to relative RMS (see definition 2), we also introduce the relative jitter, see definition 9. Using the relative jitter, we can quantify how the noise level of a predicted signal has changed with respect to the original signal.

Definition 9 (Relative jitter). Using the same notation as in definition 2, the relative jitter is defined as

$$\mathfrak{J}_{\text{rel}}(y, \delta) = \frac{\mathfrak{J}(\text{pred}(y, \delta))}{\mathfrak{J}(y)}.$$

3.3 Wavelet-based Noise Reduction

There has been very high interest in noise removal from one- or two-dimensional signals using wavelet methods. One such method which is particularly suitable to our situation has been presented in [19]. It is a non-decimated [17], discrete transform previously described in [3, 21]. It has the advantage of being shift invariant, i.e., if the first few samples are removed from our time series, the output wavelet-transformed signal remains the same.

The basic idea of the *à trous wavelet decomposition*, described in more detail in section A.1, is to iteratively convolve the input signal with an increasingly dilated wavelet function. By doing so, the original signal is transformed into a set of band-pass filtered components, so-called *scales* W_j, and the *residual* or *continuum* c_J.

3.3.1 Final noise reduction method

To summarise, the wavelet based smoothing method can be described as follows:

1. The signal is decomposed into scales $W_1, \ldots, W_J$ and the continuum c_J according to

$$c_{0,k} = y_k, \qquad c_{j+1,k} = \frac{1}{2}\left(c_{j,k-2^j} + c_{j,k}\right)$$
$$W_{j+1,k} = c_{j,k} - c_{j+1,k} \qquad\qquad (3.1)$$
$$j = 0, \ldots, J-1$$

2. Thresholding is applied to the scales W_j, $j = 1, \ldots, J$ and on the continuum c_J to compute their thresholded counterparts $\tilde{W}_n$ and $\tilde{c}_J$.
3. The smoothed signal is reconstructed by summing over the thresholded scales $\tilde{W}_n$ and continuum $\tilde{c}_J$ (refer to equation A.4).

For our application, we resort to a variation of hard thresholding and set $\tilde{W}_1 = \cdots = \tilde{W}_K = 0$ for some K which has to be selected such that the predominant part of the noise is contained in the scales $W_1, \ldots, W_K$. That this separation is indeed possible will be demonstrated using a computer generated signal in section 3.4.

The advantage of this method in comparison to Fourier analysis is the fast and simple computation—it is linear in time—and the possibility to do real time processing. Furthermore, it does not require samples from the "future" of the signal, i.e., no zero-padding or mirroring at the signal's end is necessary, which would create artefacts at the signal's end. This would be inacceptable since the end of the signal is the most important part when it comes to prediction or correlation.

3.3.2 Time Shift

A close look at equation 3.1 shows that the smoothing method resembles a multi-resolution moving average filter. Since this filtering is not centred around the current position in time, but only looks backward, the smoothed signal will be delayed in time. More specifically, removing scales one through K corresponds to a time shift of

$$\delta_K = 2^{K-1} - 0.5 \tag{3.2}$$

sampling steps for the smoothed signal. Clearly, this shift needs to be considered whenever real-time operations are to be performed on the smoothed signal. As an example, if we wish to apply smoothing to a respiratory motion trace prior to prediction, the prediction horizon has to be enlarged accordingly. This is the main reason why the smoothing method is of little use when it comes to slowly sampled signals.

Example 3. Let $y(t) = 2\sin(\pi \cdot 0.25 \cdot t)^4 + 0.3\sin(2\pi \cdot 9 \cdot t) + \nu$ and let ν be Gaussian noise with $\sigma = 0.05$ and zero mean. Let the signal be sampled at 100 Hz and let $J = 13$. This selection is somewhat arbitrary. From the above, we select $K = 4$. The resulting reconstruction and the original signal are shown in figure 3.8. Visual inspection shows that the reconstructed signal is nearly noise free. That it indeed is a very good approximation to the noise free original signal can be seen when looking at the RMS errors: $\mathrm{RMS}(\nu) = 0.05$ and

$$\mathrm{RMS}\left(y_{\{1,\dots,N-2^3\}} - \sum_{j=5}^{13} W_{j,\{1+2^3,\dots,N\}} - C_{\{1+2^3,\dots,N\}}\right) = 0.015.$$

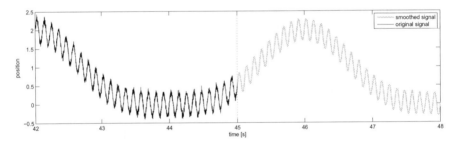

Fig. 3.8: Original signal (left, black) and smoothed signal (right, grey) from example 3. Time shift has been compensated.

The noise reduction method will also be applied to chest motion data. In this context, care must be taken to not discard relevant information: discarding all levels up to K will result in all motion be lost where relevant changes occur in less than $2^{K-1}/f$. Here, f is the sampling rate of the signal to be smoothed. In literature, different average respiratory rates for healthy adults are reported, ranging from 10 to 20 breaths per minute [5, p. 78],[22, p. 380],[23, p. 707]. Consequently, by assuming an upper bound on human respiration and requiring information at ten times this rate to be present in the smoothed signal, we find that

$$\frac{2^{K-1}}{f} \leq \frac{1}{10 f_{\max}}, \tag{3.3}$$

where f_{max} is the maximal frequency expected from respiration. The corresponding values of K for all frequencies between 10 Hz and 5 kHz, using $f_{max} = 0.5$ Hz (i.e., 30 breaths per minute) as an upper bound, are given in figure 3.9.

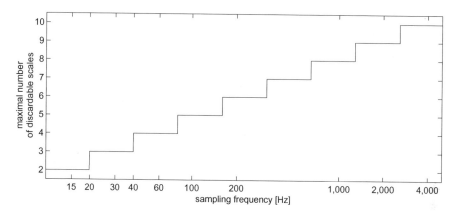

Fig. 3.9: Maximal number of discardable scales for different sampling frequencies. Note that the plot is logarithmic in the frequency axis.

In clinical practice, depending on the health and actual respiratory behaviour of the patient, other limits may be required. Using equation 3.3, however, the appropriate values can be determined easily.

3.3.3 Modified Measures for Smoothed Signals

In the context of chapter 4, we will also look at the quality of signals which have been smoothed with this method prior to prediction. To be able to do this, the notion of relative RMS (as defined in definition 2) has to be changed a little to take smoothing into account:

Definition 10 (Relative RMS for smoothed signals). Using the same notation as in definition 2, the relative RMS of a signal smoothed at level K is defined as

$$\operatorname*{RMS}_{rel}(y,r,\delta,K) = \frac{\operatorname{RMS}\left(\operatorname{pred}\left(\mathscr{W}_K(y),\delta + \delta_K\right) - r\right)}{\operatorname{RMS}\left(D(y,\delta) - r\right)}.$$

Note that here, K is the level of wavelet smoothing applied (i.e., discard the scales up to K), $\mathscr{W}_K(y)$ denotes the signal y smoothed at level K and δ_K denotes the additional delay incurred by performing wavelet smoothing at level K.

Similarly, the relative jitter of smoothed and subsequently predicted signals is defined according to definition 11.

Definition 11 (Relative jitter for smoothed signals). Using the same notation as in definition 9, the relative jitter of a signal smoothed at level K is defined as

$$\Im_{rel}(y, \delta, K) = \frac{\Im\left(\mathrm{pred}\left(\mathscr{W}_K(y), \delta + \delta_K\right)\right)}{\Im(y)}.$$

3.4 Analysing the Noise Level of Tracking Devices

As a consequence of section 3.2.2, we investigated the noise characteristics of six commercially available tracking systems (table 3.2). These systems cover a wide range of acquisition modalities (active and passive IR, visible light, magnetic) and frequencies (15 Hz to more than 4.1 kHz). The system currently used by the CyberKnife—Stryker's FP5500—is not present in this table, but its predecessor— BIG's FP5000—was tested in our lab.

Table 3.2: Tracking devices tested

Tracking Device	System Vendor	Measurement Principle	Marker Type	Max. Update Rate
A) FP5000	Boulder Innovation Group, Inc.	Triangulation, linear detectors	Active infrared	18 Hz
B) Polaris (classic)	Northern Digital Inc.	Triangulation, CCD	Active infrared	60 Hz
C) Polaris Vicra	Northern Digital Inc.	Triangulation, CCD	Passive infrared	20 Hz
D) Aurora	Northern Digital Inc.	Electromagnetic	Inductive, 5DOF	40 Hz
E) MicronTracker2 H40	Claron Technology Inc.	Triangulation, CCD	Passive visible	30 Hz
F) accuTrack 250	Atracsys LLC	Triangulation, linear detectors	Active infrared	4,111.84 Hz single LED

3.4.1 Measuring the Noise – Experimental Setup

The noise levels of the tracking systems were measured for both static targets and targets moving on a simulated respiratory motion trace. The noise reduction method explained in section 3.3 was applied to the data from the moving target study and to real respiratory motion recorded in our lab.

3.4.1.1 Static targets

For each system, a marker was tracked over six hours in our laboratory. Special attention was placed on stable and temperature-independent mounting of both the camera or field generator and the marker to be tracked. Then the systems were activated and no measurements were taken for more than six hours to allow for adaptation to the room environment. Afterwards, the lab was sealed and air-conditioned to rule out outside influence on the measurements and the measuring process was started.

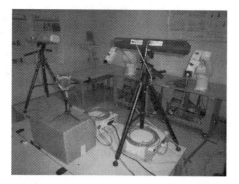

Fig. 3.10: Setup used to test the motion accuracy of NDI Polaris (classic) systems

3.4.1.2 Moving targets

To determine the noise characteristics for moving targets, the cameras/field generators were calibrated to deliver measurements in the coordinate system of the robot
carrying the marker. This was done using measurements at thirty positions randomly
selected in a sphere with radius 1 cm (this sphere encompasses the trajectory the
marker will later move on). Then the marker was moved along a trajectory in 3D
space mimicking human respiration, i.e. sinusoidal motion of different frequencies
and amplitudes in all three spatial axes, as shown in equation 3.4 and figure 3.11.

$$
\begin{aligned}
\omega &= (\omega_x, \omega_y, \omega_z)^{\mathrm{T}} = 2\pi \cdot (0.1, 0.15, 0.25)^{\mathrm{T}} \text{ Hz,} \\
a &= (a_x, a_y, a_z)^{\mathrm{T}} = (0.75, -0.3, 3)^{\mathrm{T}} \text{ mm,} \\
\mathrm{traj}(t) &= (a_x \sin(t\omega_x), a_y \sin(t\omega_y), a_z \sin(t\omega_z))^{\mathrm{T}}
\end{aligned}
\tag{3.4}
$$

That human respiratory motion indeed occurs in three axes—not only perpendicular
to the chest—has been shown before [13]. We expect the noise measured on this

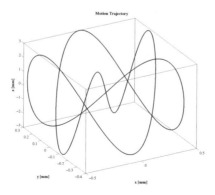

Fig. 3.11: The motion trajectory used to determine the measurement noise of a moving target

motion trajectory to be not as well behaved as the noise measured using a stationary marker. The reasons for this are:

- The motion trajectory logged by the robot may differ from the actual position of the end effector due to vibration, slack in the robot gears, and positioning inaccuracies.
- Calibration affects the measurement error which is determined by transforming the tool's position to the robot's coordinate system.
- Distortions in the measured marker geometry (more on this in section 3.5).

3.4.1.3 Acquisition of real respiratory motion

As outlined before, the smoothing method was also tested on a real respiratory motion signal. This motion trace was recorded using system (F) and an LED net [13] placed on the thorax of a male test subject (figure 3.12).

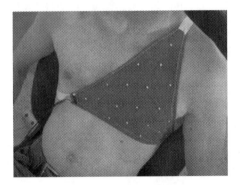

Fig. 3.12: Test subject with LED net attached

The LED net consists of 19 LEDs, resulting in a tracking rate of approximately 150 Hz for each individual LED.

3.4.2 Noise distributions measured

In this section, we will give the results of the experiments to determine the measurement noise of static and moving targets.

3.4.2.1 Static targets

We found that, for all systems tested, the noise distribution of a static target approaches a Gaussian distribution (figure 3.13 and table 3.3). The light grey line shows the distribution of Gaussian noise with the first and second moments (mean, standard deviation) of the measured signals. Although not shown here, the overall measurement accuracy depends on the actual marker position in space. But since this does not influence the general shape of the error distribution, it is disregarded. To be able to roughly compare the accuracies of the individual systems, the measurements were taken approximately at the centre of the systems' measurement volumes to obtain the best possible results. Clearly, the systems all perform very similarly with 3D RMS errors much below 0.1 mm.

Table 3.3: Distance errors of the tracking systems tested, static target

Tracking System	Standard Deviation [mm]			RMS 3D [mm]
	x	y	z	
A) FP5000	0.0048	0.0080	0.0230	0.0248
B) Polaris (classic), active	0.0072	0.0043	0.0324	0.0332
C) Polaris Vicra	0.0026	0.0028	0.0145	0.0150
D) Aurora	0.0114	0.0110	0.0186	0.0244
E) MicronTracker2 H40	0.0027	0.0070	0.0511	0.0516
F) accuTrack 250	0.0042	0.0089	0.0227	0.0248

3.4.2.2 Moving targets

The experiment using a moving target showed a sharp decrease in measurement accuracy. Nevertheless, the resulting distributions (figure 3.14) are still mostly Gaussian as long as the measurement frequency is sufficiently high. System (A), tracking at 18 Hz, shows that we suffer from some additional error which will be further investigated in section 3.5. Table 3.4 shows the resulting standard deviations and 3D RMS errors.

Table 3.4: Distance errors of the tracking systems tested, moving target, and the change in percent compared to the static target

Tracking System	Standard Deviation [mm]			RMS 3D [mm]
	x	y	z	
A) FP5000	0.0179	0.0101	0.0231	0.0311 (+25 %)
B) Polaris (classic), active	0.0204	0.0272	0.0233	0.1176 (+254 %)
C) Polaris Vicra	0.0168	0.0175	0.0917	0.0950 (+530 %)
D) Aurora	0.0856	0.0360	0.1548	0.1814 (+640 %)
E) MicronTracker2 H40	0.0442	0.1219	0.0547	0.1687 (+230 %)
F) accuTrack 250	0.0620	0.0371	0.0344	0.0817 (+229 %)

We observe that the systems' 3D accuracy has decreased substantially, by as much as 640 %, but is still below or around 0.1 mm for four of the six systems. In the case of system (B), the noise reduction method proved to be somewhat effective:

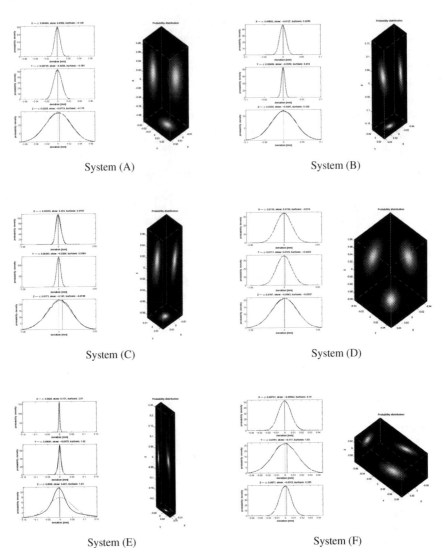

Fig. 3.13: Static error distributions of the tracking systems tested. The individual plots show
the probability density of the individual axes (in black) and the Gaussian distribution with
the same first and second moments (grey). The 3D plots show projections of the error's probability distribution.

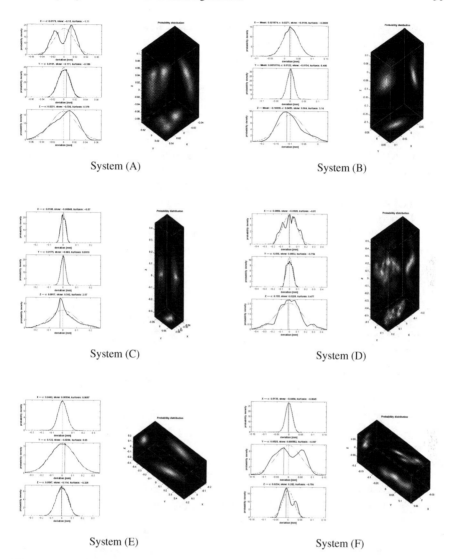

Fig. 3.14: Error distributions for moving targets. The individual plots show the probability density of the individual axes (in black) and the Gaussian distribution with the same first and second moments (grey). The 3D plots show projections of the error's probability distribution.

discarding the scales one through four resulted in the RMS of the 3D measurement error dropping from 0.1176 to 0.0677 mm, an improvement of approximately 42 %. For system (E), the RMS of the 3D measurement error drops from 0.1687 to 0.1484 mm (by 12 %) after discarding the first three scales. For system (F), removing the wavelet scales one through seven yields a reduction of about 31 % in 3D RMS error, from 0.0817 to 0.0567 mm. These numbers are given in table 3.5. In all cases, the number of scales to discard (i.e., K) was selected according to equation 3.3 and figure 3.9.

Another very important aspect of the processed signal is the fact that it has become much smoother. This smoothness is measured by the signal's jitter, see definition 8. As an example, the signal defined in equation 3.4 has a jitter of $\mathfrak{J}\left(\text{traj}(t)\right) = 3.03\frac{mm}{s}$, whereas this signal measured with system (F)—using a marker with four LEDs— has a jitter of $\mathfrak{J}(s) = 70.20\frac{mm}{s}$. Detailed values for systems (B), (E) and (F) are given in table 3.5. In fact, the jitter of the smoothed signal from all three systems is almost the same as the jitter we expect from the original signal. Figure 3.15 shows plots of the motion signal and the residual errors of the systems before (left) and after (right) smoothing.

Table 3.5: Change in jitter and RMS due to wavelet smoothing. Note that for all systems, the jitter of the smoothed signal comes close to the jitter of the original signal. K is the level of wavelet smoothing applied.

System	$\mathfrak{J}$ before smoothing	$\mathfrak{J}$ after smoothing	change in RMS	K
original	$3.03\frac{mm}{s}$	—	—	—
(B)	$3.32\frac{mm}{s}$	$2.97\frac{mm}{s}$	42 %	4
(E)	$4.40\frac{mm}{s}$	$3.01\frac{mm}{s}$	12 %	3
(F)	$70.20\frac{mm}{s}$	$3.10\frac{mm}{s}$	31 %	7

The human breathing motion recorded before (see figure 3.12) was also subjected to smoothing. Since the LED net used consists of 19 LEDs, the tracking rate for each LED was not as high as the rate for the marker used for the synthetic signal: each individual LED was tracked at approximately 150 Hz. Hence, it was not possible to perform smoothing to the same extent as with the simulated signal. Figure 3.16 shows the original signal from one LED (top row) and the smoothed signal (bottom row; scales 1 to 3 discarded). Clearly, the motion of the LED is strongest in z-direction but some motion is also present in the other axes.

In section 4.3, we will come back to this signal. It will be subject to prediction algorithms and will also be further analysed in terms of frequencies present and information removed by the smoothing method.

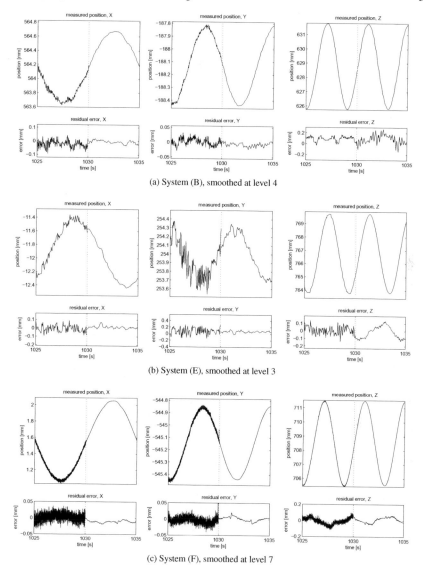

(a) System (B), smoothed at level 4

(b) System (E), smoothed at level 3

(c) System (F), smoothed at level 7

Fig. 3.15: Motion plots (top) and error signals (bottom) of a moving target. The left parts of the figures (up to the dotted vertical line) show the unprocessed signals and the right parts show the signal and the error after smoothing has been applied. Time shift has been compensated.

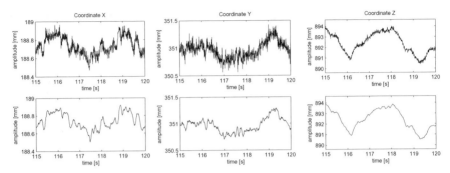

Fig. 3.16: Real breathing motion (top; see figure 3.12) and smoothed signal (bottom; scales one to three discarded). Time shift has been compensated.

3.4.3 Analysis of the results

In section 3.4.2.2 we found that the errors for systems (C) and (D) increased most in comparison to the test with a static probe. Clearly, system (C) suffers from its poor depth resolution due to the small distance between the system's two cameras and system (D) obviously struggles with moving probes in the magnetic field. This can be explained by the fact that the probe's position is measured by iteratively firing the magnetic coils in the system's field generators. And since the probe was moving, this approach clearly generates a distorted position estimate. Further analysis shows that the error signals of the IR-based active camera systems contain significant amounts of energy at the three frequencies of the motion and their multiples when tracking a marker with more than one LED. This can be explained by the fact that the error is largest when the speed of motion is highest. And since the direction of the speed is not important when it comes to the magnitude of the error, we notice significant amounts of measurement error at twice the frequency of the actual motion. This can best be seen in the spectrogram of system (A)'s measurement error (figure 3.14 and figure 3.17), since it is most vulnerable to this effect due to its low sampling rate. Clearly, we cannot expect to entirely remove this error from the signal. On

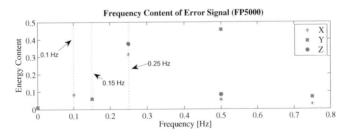

Fig. 3.17: Spectrogram of the three components of the measurement error of a moving target for system (A). All frequencies with an energy content of at least 0.01 are shown.

the other hand, random noise can be distinguished from breathing signals if the sampling rate is sufficiently high. For example, system (B) measures at 60 Hz, and from figure 3.9 we see that the first four scales can be safely removed without losing information from the breathing signal. This is supported by the fact that the main energy content of the signal measured using this system can be found in scales five or higher. For system (E), the improvement of RMS error with smooting applied was disappointing: approximately 12 %. The improvement is not higher since, as mentioned before, in each axis significant amount of energy at the frequencies of the motion in the other axes is present—albeit not as strong as in the case of system (A), see figure 3.15. This inherent error cannot be removed except at the cost of discarding too much information. Looking at figure 3.15, we see that some of the residual error after smoothing is not random but could be due to motion artefacts— i.e., the effect of frequency leakage as outlined in section 3.5 and other, unknown effects—and that the processed signal is indeed by far smoother.

3.5 Frequency Leakage

If a marker tracked using an active IR camera consists of more than one LED, the measurement accuracy when following a moving target is limited. The reason is that only one of the LEDs of the marker can be recorded per frame, resulting in a motion blurred estimate of the marker's position. Consequently, the LEDs of a moving marker will not be imaged at the same moment and therefore the measured geometry will not be the same as the real geometry (see figure 3.18). Furthermore, since the

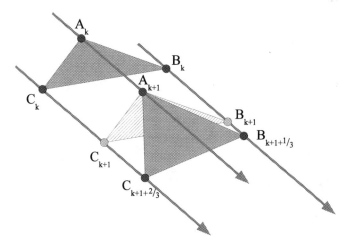

Fig. 3.18: Motion of a marker with three LEDs from one time step to the next. The image shows the original object (with LEDs A_k, B_k, and C_k), the true position at time k+1 and the actually measured pose, where LEDs B and C are measured later than LED A.

pose of a marker is usually determined by matching the measured geometry—albeit distorted—to the stored referential geometry by means of the algorithms of Horn [12] or Arun [1], the geometrical distortion will lead to incorrectly measured poses. We call this effect *frequency leakage*, since motion in one spatial axis may result in measured motion in other axes.

To analyse the impact of frequency leakage on tracking systems, we performed two motion blurring tests using the Atracsys accuTrack 250 system. This system has the ability to track single LEDs at a rate of 331.04 Hz to 4.1 kHz. Additionally, it easily supports custom-built active tools with up to 20 LEDs per tool. We used one of the tools commercially available in our motion blurring test, see figure 3.19. In the first test, the tool was attached to an adept Viper s850 robot. Hand-eye calibration was performed to have the camera deliver measurements in the robot's coordinate system. Then the tool was moved for one minute according to equation 3.5.

$$\begin{pmatrix} x(t) \\ y(t) \\ z(t) \end{pmatrix} = \begin{pmatrix} A\sin\left(2\pi f t\right) + x_0 \\ A\sin\left(2\pi f t\right) + y_0 \\ A\sin\left(2\pi f t\right) + z_0 \end{pmatrix}, \quad A = 30 \text{ mm}, \ f = 1.5 \text{ Hz} \qquad (3.5)$$

Consequently, the robot performed a linear motion on a diagonal in its coordinate system with a motion range of $2 \cdot \sqrt{3 \cdot 30^2}$ mm $= 103.92$ mm at a maximal velocity of $\sqrt{3\left(2\pi \cdot 1.5 \cdot 30\right)^2}$ mm/s $= 489.73$ mm/s.

In the second experiment, the same tool was moved by hand on a random 3D trajectory, spanning a distance of approximately 200 mm at a maximal velocity of 1,615 mm/s.

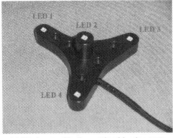

$d_{i,j}$	1	2	3	4
1	—	31.63	50.05	50.31
2	31.63	—	31.08	31.46
3	50.05	31.08	—	50.11
4	50.31	31.46	50.11	—

(a) Marker used in the motion blurring tests   (b) Distances between the individual LEDs

Fig. 3.19: Infrared marker of the accuTrack system. The marker's coordinate system is defined by LEDs one, three and four: the origin lies at LED one, the positive x-axis goes from LED one to LED three and LEDs one, three and four define the marker's x(+)-y(+)-plane.

3.5.1 Measurement Errors

We expect to see two effects: first, the distance between any two LEDs on the tool should change when the marker is moved. Second, the measured pose cannot be registered properly to the stored referential pose, resulting in a high marker registration error.

3.5.1.1 Distance errors between LEDs

We tracked the marker at a single LED measuring rate of 331.04 Hz, resulting in a time lag of 3.02 ms between the acquisition of two LEDs. Consequently, when the marker is moved as outlined before, the second LED will have moved up to 1.48 mm (robotic experiment) and 4.88 mm (manual experiment) until it is acquired. This distance will double (triple) when looking at LEDs one and three (four). In the first motion blurring test, using the marker referential geometry, we can compute the expected positions of LEDs two to four from the measured position of LED one. LED one's velocity is computed using numerical differentiation and it is assumed to be constant between two measurements to determine the position of the other LEDs. This is possible since the robot performed no rotation and hence the direction from LED one to any other LED remains fixed. According to equation 3.6, we can thus determine the anticipated position of the other LEDs.

$$\begin{pmatrix} x_i \\ y_i \\ z_i \end{pmatrix}_{\text{est}} = \begin{pmatrix} x_1 \\ y_1 \\ z_1 \end{pmatrix} + \frac{i-1}{f_{\text{acq}}} \begin{pmatrix} \dot{x}_1 \\ \dot{y}_1 \\ \dot{z}_1 \end{pmatrix} + d_{1,i}, \quad i = 2, \ldots, 4 \qquad (3.6)$$

Here, $d_{1,i}$ is the distance between LED one and LED i on the marker with respect to the robot's coordinate system, f_{acq} is the single LED acquisition frequency (331.04 Hz in our case), $(x_1, y_1, z_1)^{\text{T}}$ is the position of LED one and $(\dot{x}_1, \dot{y}_1, \dot{z}_1)^{\text{T}}$ is its speed. Subsequently, the distance between LEDs one and four was computed using both the measured and estimated positions for LED four. The distance error was computed as

$$e_k^{\text{dist}} = \left\| (x_{1,k}, y_{1,k}, z_{1,k})^{\text{T}} - (x_{4,k}, y_{4,k}, z_{4,k})^{\text{T}} \right\| - \|d_{1,4}\|$$

for the actually measured positions of LED one and four and as

$$e_k^{\text{dist,est}} = \left\| (x_{1,k}, y_{1,k}, z_{1,k})^{\text{T}} - (x_{4,k}, y_{4,k}, z_{4,k})_{\text{est}}^{\text{T}} \right\| - \|d_{1,4}\|$$

for the estimated position of LED four. In both cases, k is the temporal index of the recorded or computed time series. As expected, the estimated and actual distance errors agree very well, see figure 3.20.

It is clear that, given the numbers from figure 3.19 (b), this distance error cannot be ignored: it is up to ± 3.2 mm, or $\pm 6.4\%$, of the true distance between LEDs one and four, with a standard deviation of 2.2 mm, or 4.4 %.

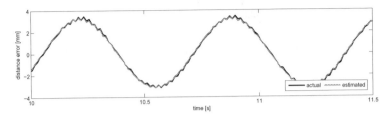

Fig. 3.20: Actual (black) and estimated grey) distance errors of the distance between LEDs one and four from the robotic motion blurring experiment.

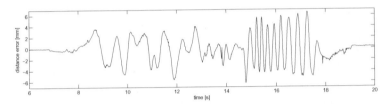

Fig. 3.21: Distance errors of the distance between LEDs one and four from the manual motion blurring experiment.

In the case of the second study, where the marker was moved by hand, it was not possible to compute an estimated distance error, since the true orientation of the marker was not known. Figure 3.21 shows the actual distance errors, being as much as 6.5 mm, or 8.0 %, with a standard deviation of 2.3 mm, or 4.6 %.

3.5.1.2 Pose errors

When measuring the LEDs, the camera not only reports the positions of the individual LEDs but, using the stored referential geometry of the marker, also computes a pose matrix describing the translation and rotation of the measured marker with respect to the camera's coordinate system. This is done using the algorithms of Horn [12] or Arun [1]. To compute the errors made using the LEDs' non-simultaneously acquired positions, we matched the referential geometry to these positions by means of the Horn algorithm. Then the average of the registration errors was computed.
Let R be the referential geometry and let P_k be the measured geometry at time k. Then the Horn algorithm determines a matrix $\mathbf{M}_k$ such that the error

$$e_k^{\text{reg}} = \sqrt{\sum_{i=1}^{4} \left\| \mathbf{M}_k \cdot R_i - P_{k,i} \right\|^2}$$

is minimised. Here, the subscript i denotes the individual points of the referential and recorded geometries. Furthermore, in the case of the robotic study, we know that the orientation of the marker with respect to the camera does not change. We can thus compare the rotation angles of the matrices $\mathbf{M}_k \cdot \mathbf{M}_0^{-1}$, where $\mathbf{M}_0$ denotes the pose matrix describing the position and orientation of the marker before the start of the motion. Let q be the Quaternion representation of the rotational part of the pose matrix $\mathbf{M}_k \cdot \mathbf{M}_0^{-1}$. Details about the conversion are given in section A.4. Then

$$q = (q_0, q_x, q_y, q_z)^{\mathrm{T}} = (\cos(\theta_k/2), \omega_k \sin(\theta_k/2))^{\mathrm{T}},$$

and consequently the rotation error can be computed as

$$e_k^{\mathrm{rot}} = 2\arccos(\theta_k). \tag{3.7}$$

Again, the results are clear: the marker registration error increases sharply from about 0.12 mm before the start of the motion to as much as 1.25 mm, depending on the current speed. Similarly, the rotation error increases from less than $0.01\,^\circ$ to as much as $3\,^\circ$. Figure 3.22 shows the graphs of these two errors.

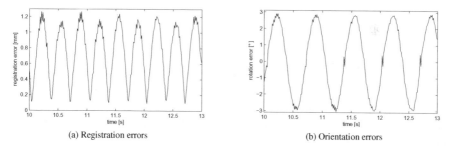

(a) Registration errors   (b) Orientation errors

Fig. 3.22: Pose errors of the motion from the robotic study

In the case of the manual motion blurring study, only the registration error could be computed, since, as mentioned before, the marker orientation was not constant during the study. Figure 3.23 shows the registration error, which was as much as 4.0 mm.

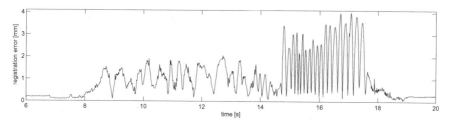

Fig. 3.23: Marker registration errors of the motion from the manual study

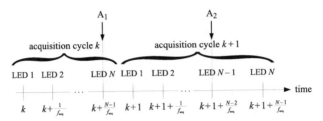

Fig. 3.24: Time axis of typical multi-LED acquisition. This shows that, to determine the positions of LEDs 1 to $N-1$ **in cycle** k **at time** $k + \frac{N-1}{f_{acq}}$**, we need to acquire the positions of these LEDs in cycle** $k + 1$**, resulting in a delay of** $\frac{N-1}{f_{acq}}$**. Position** A_1 **marks the point at which all data for the pose of the marker from cycle** k **is available (used for regular pose determination and prediction),** A_2 **marks the point at which sufficient data is available for retrospective interpolation.**

3.5.2 Compensation Strategies

There are two possible ways to compensate for the errors outlined above. Let us assume that we are currently in acqustion cycle k. Then

- we can retrospectively interpolate the positions of LEDs one to $N-1$ from cycle $k+1$ to match the timestamps of LED N in cycle k, or
- we can predict the positions of LEDs one to $N-1$ from cycle k to match the timestamps of LED N in cycle k.

This is clarified by figure 3.24. In both cases, we gain increased accuracy at some additional expense: interpolation can only be done after the next position of LEDs one to $N-1$ has been acquired, which results in an additional delay of $(N-1)/f_{acq}$—in our case, this would be 9.06 ms for $N = 4$ and $f_{acq} = 331.04$ Hz. Given that the camera system has an acquisition delay of less than 10 ms (according to the manufacturer's specifications [2] and as determined in section 3.1.1), the additional delay is not negligible. On the other hand, forecasting the position is costly in terms of computation time and possibly not as reliable as interpolation. Furthermore, since most prediction algorithms can only forecast to multiples of the sampling rate, the position signals from each LED need to be upsampled to f_{acq} to allow forecasting. We have applied both the interpolation and prediction methods to the data acquired in the motion blurring studies. Prediction was done using the toolkit described in section 4.4. The algorithm employed was the Multi-step linear methods (MULIN) algorithm (see section 4.2.3) with $n = 2$, $M = 1$ and $\mu = 0.67$. The results are convincing: for both studies, the two methods showed a significant reduction in distance and pose errors, see figure 3.25, figure 3.26 and table 3.6.

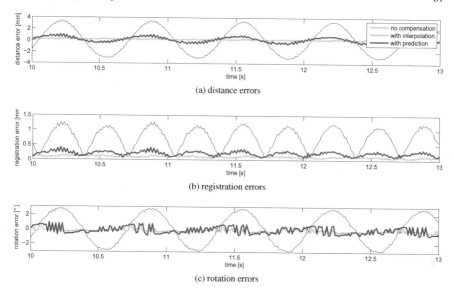

(a) distance errors

(b) registration errors

(c) rotation errors

Fig. 3.25: Marker distance and pose errors with and without compensation strategies, robot study

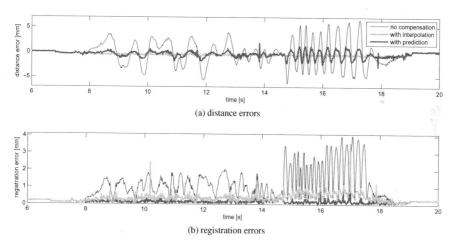

(a) distance errors

(b) registration errors

Fig. 3.26: Marker distance and pose errors with and without compensation strategies, manual study

Table 3.6: Results of the motion blurring test. Shown are the errors (standard deviation) of the distance from the first to the third LED and the RMS of the marker registration error for three possible methods.

method	robotic study			manual study	
	e^{dist}	e^{reg}	e^{rot}	e^{dist}	e^{reg}
	$(\sigma, [\%])$	(RMS, [mm])	(RMS, [°])	$(\sigma, [\%])$	(RMS, [mm])
nothing	4.40	0.91	2.09	4.61	1.36
interpolation	0.61	0.36	0.56	0.51	0.22
prediction	1.21	0.59	0.91	1.19	0.43

References

[1] Arun, K.S., Huang, T.S., Blostein, S.D.: Least-squares fitting of two 3-d point sets. IEEE Transactions on Pattern Analysis and Machine Intelligence **9**(5), 698–700 (1987)

[2] Atracsys LLC: Advanced Tracking Systems. Available online (2009). URL http://www.atracsys.com/pdfs/atracsys_tracking_systems.pdf

[3] Aussem, A., Murtagh, F.: A neuro-wavelet strategy for web traffic forecasting. Research in Official Statistics **1**(1), 65–87 (1998)

[4] Bartz, D., Bohn, S., Hoffmann, J. (eds.): Jahrestagung der Deutschen Gesellschaft für Computer- und Roboterassistierte Chirurgie, vol. 7. CURAC, Leipzig, Germany (2008)

[5] Beckett, B.S.: Illustrated Human and Social Biology. Oxford University Press, Oxford (1995)

[6] Ernst, F.: Motion compensation in radiosurgery. In: RTMART Workshop 2009. Institute for Robotics, University of Lübeck, Institute for Robotics, University of Lübeck, Lübeck, Germany (2009)

[7] Ernst, F., Bruder, R., Schlaefer, A.: Processing of respiratory signals from tracking systems for motion compensated IGRT. In: 49th Annual Meeting of the AAPM, *Medical Physics*, vol. 34, p. 2565. American Association of Physicists in Medicine, Minneapolis-St. Paul, MN, USA (2007). DOI 10.1118/1.2761413. TU-EE-A3-4

[8] Ernst, F., Bruder, R., Schlaefer, A., Schweikard, A.: Improving the quality of biomedical signal tracking using prediction algorithms. In: UKACC International Conference on CONTROL 2010, vol. 8, pp. 301–305. United Kingdom Automatic Control Council, Coventry, UK (2010)

[9] Ernst, F., Bruder, R., Schlaefer, A., Schweikard, A.: Performance measures and pre-processing for respiratory motion prediction. In: 53rd Annual Meeting of the AAPM, *Medical Physics*, vol. 38, p. 3857. American Association of Physicists in Medicine, Vancouver, CA (2011). DOI 10.1118/1.3613523. TH-C-BRC-06

[10] Ernst, F., Schlaefer, A., Schweikard, A.: Processing of respiratory motion traces for motion-compensated radiotherapy. Medical Physics **37**(1), 282–294 (2010). DOI 10.1118/1.3271684

[11] Ernst, F., Schweikard, A.: A survey of algorithms for respiratory motion prediction in robotic radiosurgery. In: S. Fischer, E. Maehle (eds.) 39. GI Jahrestagung, *Lecture Notes in Informatics*, vol. 154, pp. 1035–1043. GI, Bonner Köllen, Lübeck, Germany (2009)

[12] Horn, B.K.P.: Closed-form solution of absolute orientation using unit quaternions. Journal of the Optical Society of America A **4**(4), 629–642 (1987). DOI 10.1364/JOSAA.4.000629

[13] Knöpke, M., Ernst, F.: Flexible Markergeometrien zur Erfassung von Atmungs- und Herzbewegungen an der Körperoberfläche. In: Bartz et al. [4], pp. 15–16

[14] KUKA Robot Group: KUKA.Ethernet RSI XML 1.1. User's manual (03.05.2007)

[15] Martens, V., Ernst, F., Fränkler, T., Matthäus, L., Schlichting, S., Schweikard, A.: Ein Client-Server Framework für Trackingsysteme in medizinischen Assistenzsystemen. In: Bartz et al. [4], pp. 7–10

[16] Murphy, M.J.: Tracking moving organs in real time. Seminars in Radiation Oncology **14**(1), 91–100 (2004). DOI 10.1053/j.semradonc.2003.10.005

[17] Nason, G.P., Silverman, B.W.: Wavelets and Statistics, *Lecture Notes in Statistics*, vol. 103, chap. The stationary wavelet transform and some statistical applications, pp. 281–300. Springer (1995)

[18] Papież, L., Timmerman, R.D.: Hypofractionation in radiation therapy and its impact. Medical Physics **35**(1), 112–118 (2008). DOI 10.1118/1.2816228

[19] Renaud, O., Starck, J.L., Murtagh, F.: Wavelet-based combined signal filtering and prediction. IEEE Transactions on Systems, Man and Cybernetics, Part B: Cybernetics **35**(6), 1241–1251 (2005)

[20] Richter, L., Ernst, F., Martens, V., Matthäus, L., Schweikard, A.: Client/server framework for robot control in medical assistance systems. In: Proceedings of the 24th International Congress and Exhibition on Computer Assisted Radiology and Surgery (CARS'10), *International Journal of Computer Assisted Radiology and Surgery*, vol. 5, pp. 306–307. CARS, Geneva, Switzerland (2010)

[21] Shensa, M.J.: The discrete wavelet transform: wedding the à trous and Mallat algorithms. IEEE Transactions on Signal Processing **40**(10), 2464–2482 (1992). DOI 10.1109/78.157290

[22] Sherwood, L.: Fundamentals of Physiology: A Human Perspective. Brooks Cole, London (2006)

[23] Tortora, G.J., Anagnostakos, N.P.: Principles of Anatomy and Physiology, 6th edn. Harper-Collins, New York (1990)

Chapter 4
On the Outside: Prediction of Human Respiratory and Pulsatory Motion

As outlined in section 1.1, there will be an inevitable difference between the current target position and the position of the treatment beam. This difference originates from the latency in acquiring and computing the target position and from moving the robot. The goal clearly is to compensate for this delay and try to send the robot to a predicted position. In practice, several methods for the compensation of this delay are implemented and used clinically. These are a pattern-matching algorithm, called Zero Error Prediction (ZEP), an adaptive filter based on Least Mean Squares (LMS), a fuzzy prediction algorithm and a hybrid combination of these [35, 36].

Notation

Throughout this chapter, we will assume that y is the respiratory motion signal we wish to predict. We assume that y is uniformly sampled with sampling rate $1/\Delta t$. Consequently, y_k denotes the value of y seen at epoch k, i.e., $y_k = y((k-1)\Delta t)$. The prediction horizon is denoted by δ. A predicted value computed at epoch k will thus be denoted by $\hat{y}_{k+\delta}$. If a specific algorithm, called NAME, is used to compute a predicted value, we will write $\hat{y}_{k+\delta}^{\text{NAME}}$.

4.1 Model-based prediction methods[1]

Prediction of respiratory motion can be separated into two classes: algorithms making use of prior knowledge about the behaviour of human respiration—so-called *model-based prediction methods*—and algorithms which can in principle be applied to an arbitrary input signal—so-called *model-free prediction methods*. This section focusses on model-based prediction, while section 4.2 explains model-free prediction algorithms investigated.

---

[1] Parts of this section have been published in [30].

Assumption 4.1 *Let y be the respiratory motion signal. We assume that this signal can be modelled as a sum of finitely many sinusoidals, i.e.,*

$$y(t) = \sum_{i=1}^{N} A_i \sin\left(2\pi f_i t + \varphi_i\right). \tag{4.1}$$

Here, N is the number of frequencies used to model the signal, A_i are the corresponding amplitudes, f_i the frequencies and φ_i the phase shifts.

4.1.1 Kalman Filtering and Extended Kalman Filtering

When prediction of signals is discussed, the first approach usually mentioned is Kalman Filtering. This principle was developed in 1960 by Rudolf E. Kálmán [23] and subsequently enhanced by Kálmán and Bucy in 1961 [24]. Kalman Filter (KF) is based on the assumption of a system which can be completely described by so-called states. In general, directly observing these states is not possible and we can thus only draw conclusions about the state variables from indirect observations.

The Kalman Filter

Let k be a temporal index, let $\mathbf{x}_k$ be the state variables at epoch k. Then Kalman filtering is governed by two functions: one describes how to progress from $\mathbf{x}_{k-1}$ to $\mathbf{x}_k$, given an additional input variable $\mathbf{u}_k$ and process noise v. This function f is described in equation 4.2.

$$\mathbf{x}_k = f\left(\mathbf{x}_{k-1}, \mathbf{u}_k, k\right) + v_{k-1} \tag{4.2}$$

The second function, h, describes how the observation vector $\mathbf{z}$ is related to the states, again assuming knowledge of the additional input variable $\mathbf{u}_k$ and the observation noise ω. This function is described in equation 4.3.

$$\mathbf{z}_k = h\left(\mathbf{x}_k, \mathbf{u}_k, k\right) + \omega_k \tag{4.3}$$

Additionally, the process and observation noise are assumed to be multivariate Gaussian with zero mean. Their assumed covariances and cross covariances are given by equation 4.4.

$$
\begin{aligned}
(\mathbf{Q}_k)_{i,j} &= \mathbf{E}\left[(v_k)_i (v_k)_j^{\mathsf{T}}\right] = \delta_{ij}(\mathbf{q}_k)_i, \\
(\mathbf{R}_k)_{i,j} &= \mathbf{E}\left[(\omega_k)_i (\omega_k)_j\right] = \delta_{ij}(\mathbf{r}_k)_i, \\
\mathbf{E}\left[(v_k)_i (\omega_k)_j^{\mathsf{T}}\right] &= 0
\end{aligned}
\tag{4.4}
$$

Here, the vectors $\mathbf{r}$ and $\mathbf{q}$ need to be selected by the user. In the case of the Kalman Filter, both f and h are expected to be linear functions. Consequently, equation 4.2 and equation 4.3 are reduced to the following:

$$\mathbf{x}_k = \mathbf{F}_{k-1} \begin{pmatrix} \mathbf{x}_{k-1} \\ \mathbf{u}_k \\ k \end{pmatrix} + v_k, \quad \mathbf{z} = \mathbf{H}_k \begin{pmatrix} \mathbf{x}_k \\ \mathbf{u}_k \\ k \end{pmatrix} + \omega_k \tag{4.5}$$

To initialise the Kalman Filter, we require estimates of the system's inital states—called $\mathbf{x}_{0|0}$—and of the system's covariance matrix—called $\mathbf{P}_{0|0}$. At each epoch k, the Kalman Filter now performs the following steps:

1. Acquire a new measurement vector $\mathbf{z}_k$
2. Compute $\mathbf{F}_{k-1}$ and $\mathbf{H}_k$
3. Predict state vector

$$\mathbf{x}_{k|k-1} = f\left(\mathbf{x}_{k-1|k-1}, u_{k-1}, k-1\right)$$

4. Predict estimated covariance

$$\mathbf{P}_{k|k-1} = \mathbf{F}_{k-1}\mathbf{P}_{k-1|k-1}\mathbf{F}_{k-1}^{\mathrm{T}} + \mathbf{Q}_{k-1}$$

5. Calculate the Kalman Gain $\mathbf{K}_k$

$$\mathbf{K}_k = \mathbf{P}_{k|k-1}\mathbf{H}_k^{\mathrm{T}} \cdot \left(\mathbf{H}_k\mathbf{P}_{k|k-1}\mathbf{H}_k^{\mathrm{T}} + \mathbf{R}_k\right)^{-1}$$

6. Update state estimate

$$\mathbf{x}_{k|k} = \mathbf{x}_{k|k-1} + \mathbf{K}_k\left(\mathbf{z}_k - h\left(\mathbf{x}_{k|k-1}, \mathbf{u}_k, k\right)\right)$$

7. Update covariance matrix $\mathbf{P}$

$$\mathbf{P}_{k|k} = \left(\mathbf{1} - \mathbf{K}_k\mathbf{H}_k\right)\mathbf{P}_{k|k-1}$$

The Extended Kalman Filter

Clearly, the Kalman Filter approach is severely limited by imposing the restriction of linearity on the functions f and h. It was thus extended to the Extended Kalman Filter (EKF) to allow modelling arbitrary functions f and h (as long as they are continuously partially differentiable). This is achieved by replacing $\mathbf{F}_{k-1}$ and $\mathbf{H}_k$ by the Jacobians of f and h:

$$\mathbf{F}_{k-1} = \frac{\partial f}{\partial \mathbf{x}}\bigg|_{\mathbf{x}_{k-1|k-1}, \mathbf{u}_{k-1}, k-1}, \qquad \mathbf{H}_k = \frac{\partial h}{\partial \mathbf{x}}\bigg|_{\mathbf{x}_{k|k-1}, \mathbf{u}_k, k} \tag{4.6}$$

In the case of strong nonlinearities, however, the filter will produce inadequate results due to the above linearisation process.

Predicting Respiratory Motion using the Extended Kalman Filter

We now present a new application of the EKF to respiratory motion prediction, first published in [30]. To this end, we come back to the description of respiratory motion introduced in assumption 4.1. This model is slightly expanded to be able to deal with signal drift:

$$y(t) = c_0 + c_1 t + \sum_{i=1}^{N} A_i \sin(2\pi f_i t + \varphi_i) \tag{4.7}$$

By comparing this model to the Kalman filter equations (equation 4.2 and equation 4.3), the required components of the EKF model can now be determined:

- State variables. We can define the states of the model as a vector containing the amplitudes, frequencies and phase shifts of the sinusoidals used, i.e.,

$$\mathbf{x}_k = ((A_k)_1, (f_k)_1, (\varphi_k)_1, \dots, (A_k)_N, (f_k)_N, (\varphi_k)_N, c_0, c_1)^{\mathrm{T}}.$$

- State transition. The state transition function f can be modelled very simply by assuming that the frequencies and amplitudes only drift randomly, i.e.,

$$(A_k)_i = (A_{k-1})_i + (v_{k-1})_{3(i-1)+1}, \quad (f_k)_i = (f_{k-1})_i + (v_{k-1})_{3(i-1)+2},$$

whereas the change of the phase shift also depends on the last frequency state:

$$(\varphi_k)_i = (\varphi_{k-1})_i + 2\pi (f_{k-1})_i \Delta t + (v_{k-1})_{3i}.$$

Consequently,

$$(\mathbf{x}_k)_i = (\mathbf{x}_{k-1})_i + \delta_{i \bmod 3,0} 2\pi (\mathbf{x}_{k-1})_{i-1} \Delta t + (v_{k-1})_i, \quad i = 1, \dots, 3N \tag{4.8}$$

where $\delta_{i \bmod 3,0} = 1$ if and only if $i \equiv 0 \bmod 3$ and 0 otherwise. Similarly, the coefficient c_1 only changes randomly while the change of c_0 also depends on the previous value of c_1:

$$c_{0,k} = c_{0,k-1} + c_{1,k-1} \Delta t + (v_{k-1})_{3N+1}, \quad c_{1,k} = c_{1,k-1} + (v_{k-1})_{3N+2}$$

- Observation function. The observation function can now be expressed in terms of the state variables:

$$\mathbf{z}_k = (\mathbf{x}_k)_{3N+1} + (\mathbf{x}_k)_{3N+2} \Delta t + \sum_{i=0}^{N-1} (\mathbf{x}_k)_{3i+1} \sin\left(2\pi (\mathbf{x}_k)_{3i+2} \Delta t + (\mathbf{x}_k)_{3i+3}\right) + \omega_k \tag{4.9}$$

Here, the additional input $\mathbf{u}_k = \Delta t$. Although the state transition function (see equation 4.8) is linear in $\mathbf{x}$, the observation function (see equation 4.9) is not. Consequently, we must use the EKF to model this problem. The Jacobians used are given in equation 4.11 and equation 4.10.

$$(\mathbf{F}_k)_{i,j} = \begin{cases} 1 & \text{if } i = j \\ 2\pi\Delta t & \text{if } i = j + 1 \text{ and } i \equiv 0 \bmod 3 \\ \Delta t & \text{if } i = 3N + 1 \text{ and } j = 3N + 2 \\ 0 & \text{otherwise} \end{cases} \tag{4.10}$$

$$(\mathbf{H}_k)_i = \begin{cases} \sin\left(2\pi(\mathbf{x}_k)_{i+1}\Delta t + (\mathbf{x}_k)_{i+2}\right) & \text{if } i \equiv 1 \bmod 3 \text{ and } i \leq 3N \\ 2\pi\Delta t\,(\mathbf{x}_k)_{i-1}\cos\left(2\pi(\mathbf{x}_k)_i\Delta t + (\mathbf{x}_k)_{i+1}\right) & \text{if } i \equiv 2 \bmod 3 \text{ and } i \leq 3N \\ (\mathbf{x}_k)_{i-2}\cos\left(2\pi(\mathbf{x}_k)_{i-1}\Delta t + (\mathbf{x}_k)_i\right) & \text{if } i \equiv 0 \bmod 3 \text{ and } i \leq 3N \\ 1 & \text{if } i = 3N + 1 \\ \Delta t & \text{if } i = 3N + 2 \end{cases}$$

$$\tag{4.11}$$

Here, $i, j = 1, \ldots, 3N + 2$, $\mathbf{H}_k^{\mathrm{T}} \in \mathbb{R}^{3N+2}$, and $\mathbf{F}_k \in \mathbb{R}^{(3N+2)\times(3N+2)}$. It is now possible to build the Extended Kalman Filter needed for frequency, amplitude, and phase tracking of respiratory motion. Actual prediction, with a prediction horizon of δ samples, say, is done according to equation 4.12.

$$\hat{y}_{k+\delta}^{\mathrm{EKF}} = (\mathbf{x}_k)_{3N+1} + (\mathbf{x}_k)_{3N+2}(1+\delta)\Delta t +$$
$$+ \sum_{i=0}^{N-1}(\mathbf{x}_k)_{3i+1}\sin\left(2\pi(\mathbf{x}_k)_{3i+2}(1+\delta)\Delta t + (\mathbf{x}_k)_{3i+3}\right) \tag{4.12}$$

Initialisation and Parameter Selection

Let y be the time series of respiratory motion we want to predict. To actually use the EKF, several parameters need to be selected:

- N, the number of sinusoidals used in assumption 4.1
- f, A and φ, the initial values of the frequencies, amplitudes and phase offsets
- $\mathbf{q}$, the covariance vector of the process noise
- $\mathbf{r}$, the covariance vector of the observation noise
- $\mathbf{p}$, the initial value for the estimated covariance matrix $\mathbf{P}$

To get initial values for f, A and φ, we select a training window size M and perform a Fast Fourier Transform (FFT) on the samples $y_1, \ldots, y_M$. Using this transform, the frequencies $f_1, \ldots, f_N$ with the highest power $|Y(f_i)|$ are selected and the corresponding amplitudes A and phase offsets φ are extracted. This is done by using a thresholded extremal search, see listing E.3 in appendix E. Selection of the observation noise covariance vector $\mathbf{r}$ should depend on the tracking modality used (to incorporate its measurement noise) and on the confidence placed in the model from assumption 4.1. Selecting proper values for $\mathbf{q}$, the process noise covariance vector, depends on the behaviour of the patient's respiratory motion. The more fluctuation is seen, the larger the values in $\mathbf{q}$ should be. $\mathbf{p}$ is selected as 0.1.

Example 4. Let y be a simulated respiratory motion signal (see appendix D) using $A = 2$, $f = 0.2$, $e_1 = 4$, $e_2 = 6$ and $t = (0, 0.01, \ldots, 400)^T$. The modification parameters were $\delta_A = 0.1$, $\delta_b = 0.1$, $\delta_B = 0.3$, $N_B = 20$, $\delta_T = 0.1$, $\sigma = 0.015$. Using $M = 1500$, this signal was predicted using the EKF method presented above. The prediction horizon was set to 150 ms, i.e., $\delta = 15$. The number of frequencies, N, was set to 3. The state error estimate was set to 0.001, the measurement error estimate was set to 0.1. The initial covariance estimate was set to 0.1. Using these settings, the predictor achieved the following results: RMS = 0.039 mm, down from 0.162 mm (RMS$_{rel}$ = 0.240), jitter $\mathfrak{J} = 0.960$, down from 1.892 ($\mathfrak{J}_{rel} = 0.507$). The signal, the prediction result and the states are shown in figure 4.1. Additionally, the state and measurement error estimates were evaluated on a 200×200 element grid on $[0, 1] \times [0, 1]$. The resulting RMS errors are shown in figure 4.2. Unfortunately, it becomes clear that, although the area of stability is quite large, selecting proper parameters is difficult: even within the area of very low RMS error, there are peaks with very large errors. This makes parameter selection for the algorithm very hard.

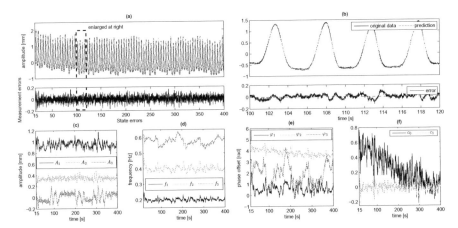

Fig. 4.1: This figure shows the signal from example 4 (graphs (a) and (b), top, black curves), the prediction output using three frequencies (graphs (a) and (b), top, grey curves), the prediction error (graphs (a) and (b), bottom) and the states as tracked by the filter (graphs (c), (d), (e) and (f)). Graph (b) is an enlargement of the dotted rectangle in graph (a). Note that for graphs (e) and (f), the phases and the coefficient c_0 have been unwrapped.

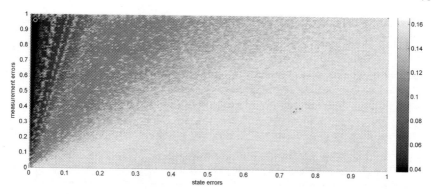

Fig. 4.2: This graphs shows the dependency of the RMS error on the EKF prediction algorithm's main parameters, the state and measurement errors. It is clear that, while a region with low error is clearly visible, the error surface is not smooth. Parameter selection for the EKF algorithm can thus be difficult. In this example, the minimal RMS of 0.0378 (RMS$_{rel}$ = 0.234) was obtained using measurement errors of 0.9598 and state errors of 0.0151, marked with a white circle. The resulting jitter is $\mathfrak{J} = 1.008$ ($\mathfrak{J}_{rel} = 0.533$).

4.2 Model-free Prediction Methods[2]

As outlined before (see section 4.1), we now focus on prediction algorithms which work without assuming prior knowledge about the signal we wish to predict.

4.2.1 Autoregressive approaches

Many algorithms for respiratory motion prediction are based on the general assumption of a local Autoregressive Moving Average (ARMA) model, some with variations thereof [11, 15–17, 28, 31, 38]. Since the time series stemming from human respiration closely resembles a superposition of sinusoidal signals, this assumption is reasonable. The autoregressive property is described in definition 12.

Definition 12 (Autoregressive processes). Let s be a uniformly sampled signal and let n be a positive integer. We say that s is an AR(n,M)-process if there is an integer M such that, when the last M values $s_{k-M+1}, \ldots, s_k$ of the signal s are known, there are weights $w = (w_1, \ldots, w_M)^{\mathrm{T}}$ satisfying $y_m = w^{\mathrm{T}} u_{m-n}$ for all $m \geq k + n$. Here, $u_{m-n} = (s_{m-n-M+1}, \ldots, s_{m-n})^{\mathrm{T}}$.

---

[2] Parts of this section have been published in [10, 11, 14–18]

4.2.1.1 Least Mean Squares and normalised Least Mean Squares prediction

One way of learning the weights of an autoregressive process is the LMS algorithm [20, 22, 40], which has been used for a long time in time series prediction and signal analysis. It was invented in 1960 by Bernard Widrow and Marcian Edward Hoff [40]. This algorithm is currently used clinically in Accuray's Synchrony system and is included in this work as a baseline for the development of other, more sophisticated approaches.

For this method, we need to select a proper signal history length M. Then the initial values w_1 to $w_{M+\delta}$ for the LMS weights are set to

$$w_1 = w_2 = \cdots = w_{M+\delta} = \mathbf{e}_M = (0, \ldots, 0, 1)^\mathrm{T} \in \mathbb{R}^M.$$

Next, for each $k \geq M$, the signal history u_k (also called "tap input vector") is built as

$$u_k = \left(u_{k,1}, \ldots, u_{k,M} \right)^\mathrm{T} = \left(y_{k-M+1}, \ldots, y_k \right)^\mathrm{T}.$$

Using these variables, the prediction output can be computed:

$$\hat{y}_{k+\delta}^{\mathrm{LMS}} = w_k^\mathrm{T} u_k, \quad k \geq M.$$

And finally, for $k \geq M + \delta$, the weights are updated as

$$w_{k+1} = w_k + \mu \left(\hat{y}_k^{y_k - \mathrm{LMS}} \right) u_{k-\delta}, \tag{4.13}$$

where μ is the algorithm's learning factor.

For stationary signals, the LMS algorithm is known to perfectly adapt to the system if the parameters μ and M are chosen properly. Note that this method is a slightly modified version of the algorithm outlined in [22, Ch. 5.2]. Difficulties arise from the fact that in the update term for the weight vector w large signal values lead to a larger correction term, i.e., when provided with two differently scaled versions (with respect to amplitude) of a signal, the algorithm produces different results.

To improve the convergence properties of the LMS algorithm (i.e., to make it independent from scaling and increase the rate of convergence), Normalised Least Mean Squares (nLMS) algorithms are used [7]. The only difference to the LMS algorithm is the way the weights are updated. To compute the nLMS prediction, we need to introduce a new parameter, $p \in \mathbb{N} \cup \{\infty\}$, which corresponds to the norm used, i.e., a whole family of algorithms, the nLMS_p algorithms, is formed. Then, instead of using $u_{k-\delta}$ as error correction term, a more generic formulation is used. Equation 4.13 is replaced by

$$w_{p,k+1} = w_{p,k} + \mu \left(\hat{y}_k^{y_k - \mathrm{nLMS}p} \right) f_{p,k-\delta}. \tag{4.14}$$

The parameter p thus governs the way the error correction term $f_{p,k}$ is computed, which is defined as follows:

$$\left(f_{p,k}\right)_i = \frac{|u_{k,i}|^{p-1}\operatorname{sgn}\left(u_{k,i}\right)}{\|u_k\|_p^p}, \, p \in \mathbb{N}$$

$$\left(f_{\infty,k}\right)_i = \frac{\delta_{i,l}}{u_{k,l}}, \quad l = \max_{j=1,\dots,M} |u_{k,j}|,$$

(4.15)

where $\delta_{i,j}$ is the Kronecker delta. In our case, we will mostly consider the special case of $p = 2$ (i.e., normalisation with respect to the Euclidean norm), hence the algorithm reduces to the following:

$$\hat{y}_{k+\delta}^{\text{nLMS2}} = w_{2,k}^T u_k$$
$$w_{2,k+1} = w_{2,k} + \mu \left(\hat{y}_k^{\text{nLMS2}} - y_k\right) f_{2,k-\delta} =$$
$$= w_{2,k} + \mu \left(\hat{y}_k^{\text{nLMS2}} - y_k\right) \frac{u_{k-\delta}}{\alpha + \|u_{k-\delta}\|_2^2}$$

(4.16)

To avoid division by zero, a small parameter α (typically 10^{-4}) is introduced in the denominator of the error term $f_{p,k}$ in equation 4.15. This was also done in equation 4.16. Again, this equation is merely a slightly modified version of [7].

Example 5. Let us come back to the signal from example 4. Prediction of this signal was performed using the nLMS$_p$-algorithms for $p = 1,2,\dots,11$ and $p = \infty$, $M = 1,\dots,100$ and $\mu = 0,0.005,\dots,0.1$. The results are shown in figure 4.3 and figure 4.4. It can be observed that, with increasing p, the minimal RMS value decreases, the corresponding values of M increase and of μ decrease. Additionally, the complexity of the error surface increases. Especially for $p = \infty$, we can observe the existence of multiple local minima. This is a big problem for any optimisation process trying to determine optimal parameters.

Similar behaviour is observed when the same evaluation was performed on a real respiratory motion signal (7,781 samples, 26 Hz sampling rate). The results are shown in figure 4.5 and figure 4.6. Here, however, even further improvement is observed for using $p = \infty$, while the error surface looks somewhat more reasonable.

4.2.1.2 Recursive Least Squares prediction

Another possible way to determine the weights of an autoregressive process is the Recursive Least Squares (RLS) algorithm [22, Ch. 9]. Haykin calls this algorithm 'a natural extension of the methods of least [mean] squares'. The main difference between the LMS and the RLS algorithms is the way the weights are updated. While the LMS algorithms are known to be sensitive to changes in the spread of the signal's ensemble-average correlation matrix **R**, the RLS algorithm circumvents this problem by using a more complex learning term: the scalar value μ of the LMS algorithms is replaced by a time-varying gain value. This algorithm was, in the slightly extended version outlined below, first applied to respiratory motion prediction in [16].

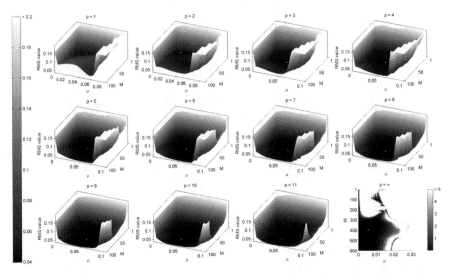

Fig. 4.3: RMS error of nLMS prediction of the signal from example 5 using different values for p, M and μ. The minimal RMS values are marked with white dots. The RMS error decreases with increasing p while the structure of the error surface becomes more and more complex. Minimal RMS is 0.0397 mm ($p = 12$, $M = 73$ and $\mu = 0.0421$).

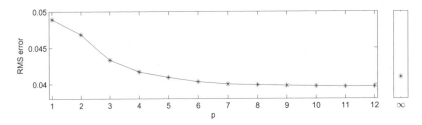

Fig. 4.4: Minimal RMS errors of the nLMS$_p$ algorithms, simulated signal.

Consequently, the possibility to use this algorithm to predict human respiration has also been investigated. Let $\hat{Y}_1,\ldots,\hat{Y}_{M+\delta-1} = y_1$. Then the RLS algorithm works as follows:

1. Select a signal history length M, a forgetting factor λ, and an initial estimate ε for the autocorrelation matrix $\mathbf{P}$
2. Initialise the tap input weight vector

$$w_1 = w_2 = \cdots = w_M = [0,\ldots,0]^{\mathrm{T}} \in \mathbb{R}^M$$

and the autocorrelation matrix

$$\mathbf{P}_1 = \varepsilon^{-1}\mathbf{I} \in \mathbb{R}^{M \times M},$$

where $\mathbf{I}$ is the identity matrix.

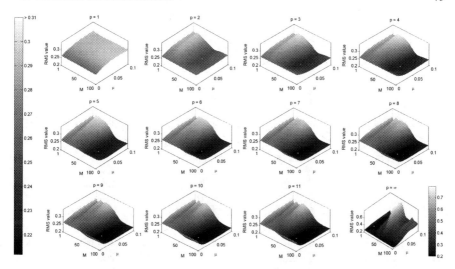

Fig. 4.5: RMS error of nLMS prediction on a real respiratory motion signal using different values for p, M and μ. The minimal RMS values are marked with white dots. Just as in figure 4.3, the RMS error decreases with increasing p while the structure of the error surface becomes more and more complex. Minimal RMS is 0.200 mm ($p = \infty$, $M = 4$ and $\mu = 0.0368$).

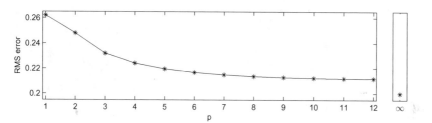

Fig. 4.6: Minimal RMS errors of the nLMS$_p$ algorithms, real respiratory signal.

3. For each sample $k \geq M$, compute

- the signal history

$$u_k = [y_k, y_{k-1}, \ldots, y_{k-M+1}]^{\mathrm{T}},$$

- the previous prediction error

$$\xi_k = y_k - \hat{Y}_k,$$

- the gain value

$$g_k = \frac{\mathbf{P}_k u_k}{\lambda + u_k^{\mathrm{T}} \mathbf{P}_k u_k},$$

- the updated autocorrelation matrix

$$\mathbf{P}_{k+1} = \lambda^{-1} \left(\mathbf{P}_k - g_k u_k^{\mathrm{T}} \mathbf{P}_k \right),$$

- and the new weights

$$w_{k+1} = w_k + g_k \xi_k.$$

4. The predicted value can then be computed as

$$\hat{Y}_{k+\delta} = w_k^T u_k.$$

Since the signals from human respiration measured with optical tracking systems are subject to system noise, we modify the RLS algorithm by adding an exponential smoothing parameter, μ, to deal with this problem.

5. To deal with signal noise, the actual prediction value is computed as

$$\hat{y}_{k+\delta}^{RLS} = (1 - \mu)\hat{Y}_{k+\delta} + \mu \hat{y}_{k+\delta-1}^{RLS}.$$

In [22, p. 463], Haykin also states that 'the rate of convergence of the RLS algorithm is typically an order of magnitude faster than that of the LMS algorithm' and that this applies to 'a stationary environment with the exponential weighting factor $\lambda = 1$'.

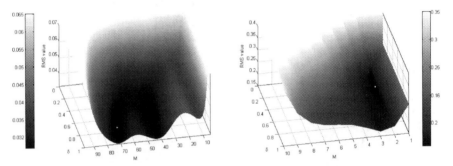

Fig. 4.7: Error surface of the RLS algorithm for different values of M and δ. Left: results for the simulated signal from example 4. Right: results for the real respiratory signal.

Example 6. We come back to the signals used in example 5. By using a grid search, it was determined that for both the simulated and the real motion signal, λ should be approximately equal to one. This is in nice correspondence with the assumption of stationarity (see assumption 4.1) and Haykin's statement. For both signals, μ was selected to be 0.15, it was also observed that the influence of moderate changes in μ on the prediction performance was very small. We thus used $\mu = 0.1$ and $\lambda = 1.0016$ on both signals. The selection of M and δ, however, is more interesting. In the case of the simulated signal, we can once more observe that the error surface sports multiple local minima; for the real signal, however, $M = 2$ is clearly optimal. The minimal RMS values are 0.0319 mm (simulated signal, $\delta = 0.740$, $M = 68$) and 0.1583 mm (real signal, $\delta = 0.240$, $M = 2$). The error surfaces are shown in figure 4.7.

4.2.1.3 Wavelet-based multiscale autoregression

In [32, 33] it has been proposed to perform signal prediction using its à trous wavelet decomposition. In section 3.3 and section A.1, this decomposition method has been described in great detail. The applicability of this method and the algorithm outlined below, with some tailoring to the specific application, was presented in [11].

Let us assume that we have computed the signal's wavelet decomposition up to level J. We thus get $J+1$ bands representing the signal: $W_1,\ldots,W_J$, the wavelet scales, and c_J, the residual, such that $y_k = W_{1,k} + \cdots + W_{J,k} + c_{J,k}$. This decomposition now allows us to perform prediction on each individual band.

We now assume the AR(2^{a_j})-property on all bands W_j and the AR($2^{a_{J+1}}$)-property on c_J. Selecting these regression depths a_j is done empirically by setting them according to equation 4.17.

$$a_j = 15 \left\lceil \frac{W_j^{\mathrm{T}} W_j}{(y - c_J)^{\mathrm{T}}(y - c_J)} \right\rceil, \quad a_{J+1} = 2 \tag{4.17}$$

Furthermore, assuming knowledge of the proper weight vectors $w_j^{(k)}$, $j = 1,\ldots,J+1$, for each band, we can state the Multiscale Autoregression (MAR) forecasting formula:

$$\hat{y}_{k+\delta}^{\mathrm{MAR}} = \sum_{j=1}^{J} \left(w_j^{(k)}\right)^{\mathrm{T}} \tilde{W}_{j,k} + \left(w_{J+1}^{(k)}\right)^{\mathrm{T}} \tilde{c}_k \tag{4.18}$$

Here, the vectors $\tilde{W}_{j,k}$ and $\tilde{c}_k$ take the role of the vector u_n (the signal history) in the LMS, nLMS, and RLS algorithms and are computed as

$$
\begin{aligned}
\tilde{W}_{j,k} &= \left(W_{j,k-2^j \cdot 0}, W_{j,k-2^j \cdot 1}, \ldots, W_{j,k-2^j(a_j-1)}\right)^{\mathrm{T}}, \\
\tilde{c}_k &= \left(c_{J,k-2^J \cdot 0}, c_{J,k-2^J \cdot 1}, \ldots, c_{J,k-2^J(a_{J+1}-1)}\right)^{\mathrm{T}}.
\end{aligned}
\tag{4.19}
$$

The correct values for the weight vectors w_j are not known, however, and need to be adaptively learned. This is done by least mean squares fitting to the last M signal steps. Let

$$l_t = \left(\tilde{W}_{1,t}^{\mathrm{T}}, \ldots, \tilde{W}_{J,t}^{\mathrm{T}}, \tilde{c}_t^{\mathrm{T}}\right)^{\mathrm{T}}.$$

Then we can define the matrix $\mathbf{B}_k$ as

$$\mathbf{B}_k = (l_{k-\delta}, \ldots, l_{k-\delta-M+1})^{\mathrm{T}}.$$

If we now define the weight vector $w_k = \left(\left(w_1^{(k)}\right)^{\mathrm{T}}, \ldots, \left(w_{J+1}^{(k)}\right)^{\mathrm{T}}\right)^{\mathrm{T}}$ and the signal history vector $s_k = (y_k, \ldots, y_{k-M+1})^{\mathrm{T}}$, it becomes possible to compute the weight vector w_{k+1} corresponding to the next epoch as

$$w_{k+1} = \left(\mathbf{B}_k^{\mathrm{T}} \mathbf{B}_k\right)^{-1} s_k. \tag{4.20}$$

This completes the description of the Wavelet-based Multiscale Autoregression (wMAR) algorithm. Clearly, the use of the matrix $\left(\mathbf{B}_k^{\mathrm{T}} \mathbf{B}_k\right)^{-1}$ is not very wise since the matrix of the normal equation (i.e., $\mathbf{B}_k$) used in equation 4.20 might not be regular. We have thus improved the algorithm to cope with irregularity. This is done by replacing $\left(\mathbf{B}_k^{\mathrm{T}} \mathbf{B}_k\right)^{-1}$ by the Moore-Penrose pseudo inverse of $\mathbf{B}_k$. This does not alter the results whenever the rank of $\mathbf{B}_k$ is maximal, it only improves numerical stability.

Additionally, looking at the MAR update equation reveals that for each point in time there is a maximum number of past observations which influence the prediction outcome. It is, however, possible that information not contained in the signal history (the vectors $\tilde{W}_{j,k}$ and $\tilde{c}_k$) still influences the future of the time series. To include this information in the prediction, we introduce an exponential averaging parameter μ and modify the wMAR method as follows, creating the Wavelet-based multiscale LMS prediction (wLMS) algorithm:

$$\hat{y}_{k+\delta}^{\text{wLMS}} = \sum_{j=1}^{J} \left(w_j^{(k)}\right)^{\mathrm{T}} \tilde{W}_{j,k} + \left(w_{J+1}^{(k)}\right)^{\mathrm{T}} \tilde{c}_k \tag{4.21}$$

$$w_{k+1} = (1-\mu)w_k + \mu \mathbf{B}_k^+ s_k, \quad \mu \in [0,1], \quad k \geq \delta + M$$

Here, w_k and s_k are as before, $w_1, \ldots, w_{M+\delta} = (0, \ldots, 0)^{\mathrm{T}}$. Additionally, the symbol $^+$ denotes the Moore-Penrose pseudo inverse of a matrix. Small values of μ correspond to a prediction with high confidence in the past while large values correspond to high confidence in recent observations. Note that with the introduction of μ there is no explicit signal history length and that setting $\mu = 1$ will yield the results of the original wMAR algorithm.

Example 7. Using the motion data described in examples 4 and 5, the wLMS algorithm was evaluated for $J = 1, \ldots, 9$, $M = 1, \ldots, 150$ and $\mu \in [0,1]$. The error plots for the simulated signal are shown in figure 4.8, the plots for the real signal are shown in figure 4.9. Optimal parameters resulted in an RMS of 0.0479 (for $J = 7$, $M = 121$ and $\mu = 1$) on the simulated signal and an RMS of 0.1494 (for $J = 3$, $M = 199$ and $\mu = 0.0204$) on the real signal.

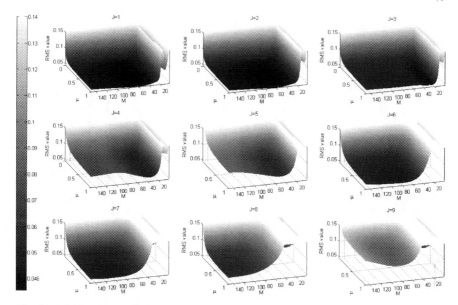

Fig. 4.8: RMS errors of the wLMS algorithm for different values of J, M and μ, simulated signal. Minimal RMS of 0.0456 was obtained using $J = 2$, $M = 57$ and $\mu = 1$.

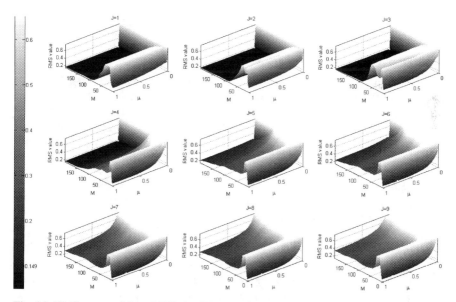

Fig. 4.9: RMS errors of the wLMS algorithm for different values of J, M and μ, real signal. Minimal RMS of 0.1494 was obtained using $J = 3$, $M = 199$ and $\mu = 0.0204$.

4.2.2 A Fast Lane Approach to LMS Prediction

Although both the LMS and the nLMS algorithms have been considered as predictors for respiratory motion signals in image-guided radiotherapy (section 4.2.1.1), there is a severe pitfall: the major problem of all algorithms of this family is the difficult task of selecting the learning parameter μ and the signal history length M. We saw that especially the selection of μ is crucial since slightly off-optimum values will cause the LMS algorithm to diverge. Since the best value of μ is not known (it depends, among other factors, on the eigenvalues of the autocorrelation matrix of the tap inputs [22, p. 306]), the usual approach of selecting μ is based on experience and guesswork.

This problem was shown in figure 4.5.

A different approach, which currently is the only viable, although not always feasible, way to use LMS-based prediction on signals of unknown characteristics, is to perform a grid search for the optimal parameters based on the first few hundred (or thousand) sampling points. Then the parameters determined on this small subset of the signal are used for the prediction process on the remainder of the signal. This method, though, has an inherent problem: the predictor is fitted to the first minute or two of breathing after the patient has been positioned for treatment. This may lead to unforeseeable errors in the performance of the prediction algorithm since it has been observed at Georgetown University Hospital that patients change their breathing pattern once they get familiar with the treatment situation and start to calm down. Nevertheless, the approach is computationally feasible: if about 96 seconds of breathing data are available (in the case of our data, this corresponds to about 2,500 sampling points), using a grid search to optimise both μ and M takes approximately one second on a Pentium 4 with 2.80 GHz running ubuntu Linux.

Another problem is the fact that the autocorrelation matrix of the tap inputs may change. As a result, when the patient falls asleep and his breathing behaviour changes, a formerly stable algorithm may start to diverge. That this can actually happen is shown in the following example.

Example 8. We performed a test on two sets of simulated data, one with changing frequency and one with changing amplitude. The first part of both test signals is a sinusoidal of 0.1 Hz (amplitude 2 mm), the second part of the first signal is a sinusoidal of 0.4 Hz (amplitude 2 mm), the second part of the second signal is a sinusoidal of 0.1 Hz (amplitude 4 mm). All test signals are sampled at 50 Hz. The resulting signals were corrupted by random Gaussian noise with a standard deviation of 0.04 mm and zero mean. Then the nLMS$_2$ algorithm was applied to the signals using $\mu = 0.2$, $M = 50$ and a prediction horizon of five samples. Figure 4.10 shows the results.

Clearly, the algorithm is able to adapt well to the first part of the signals, yielding an RMS error of 0.13 mm. But when the signal's characteristics change at sampling point 25,000 (where the autocorrelation matrix of the tap inputs changes as well, see table 4.1), the nLMS$_2$ algorithm breaks down in both cases: the prediction drifts away from the correct value.

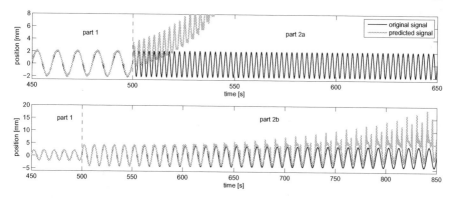

Fig. 4.10: Simulated signal with changing characteristics showing the breakdown of nLMS$_2$ prediction. Top: changing frequency, bottom: changing amplitude

Table 4.1: Largest eigenvalues of the autocorrelation matrices of the two signals with changing characteristics (see figure 4.10) in their second part (50 tap inputs). Part 1 has $f = 0.1$ Hz, $a = 2$ mm, Part 2a has $f = 0.4$ Hz, $a = 2$ mm, Part 2b has $f = 0.1$ Hz, $a = 4$ mm.

part 1	part 2a	part 2b
48.34989	30.82468	48.37823
1.60580	19.11554	1.60621
0.00087	0.00091	0.00022
0.00087	0.00091	0.00022
⋮	⋮	⋮

Clinical experience at Georgetown University Hospital has shown that when a patient falls asleep the change in respiration frequency may be less pronounced. On the other hand, significant changes in amplitude and signal shape have been observed: the exhalation phase and the rest period at maximum exhale both become longer, and the breathing amplitude increases. [6]

To overcome these problems, a new algorithm, first presented in [10], is introduced. We propose to simultaneously evaluate the prediction algorithm using different learning coefficients and signal history lengths and use the one which promises the best results. This is done by selecting initial estimates μ_0 and M_0. Then, $3N$ predictors (N odd) using the step sizes $\sigma\mu_0, \sigma\mu_0 + 2(\mu_0 - \sigma\mu_0)/(N-1), \ldots, (2-\sigma)\mu_0$ for some $\sigma \in]0, 1[$ and signal history lengths $M_0 - 1, M_0, M_0 + 1$ are initialised. All these $3N$ predictors are then evaluated in parallel, while the initial predictor (i.e., the one with $\mu = \mu_0$ and $M = M_0$) is used for prediction. After some time, the performance of all these predictors is compared and the process is restarted, seeding with the newly found "best" values for μ and M. We call this method the Fast Lane Approach (FLA), since we evaluate several parallel lanes of the algorithm (three so-called M-lanes and N so-called μ-lanes per M-lane) and switch between them trying to obtain the best possible prediction. This method is visualised in figure 4.11.

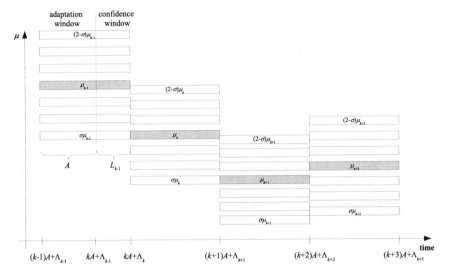

Fig. 4.11: Schematic overview of the Fast Lane Approach. The grey boxes stand for the currently used algorithm. This graphic only shows the evaluation process for one M-lane.

The algorithm is now outlined in more detail:

1. Select a starting value for μ_0, an odd number of desired parallel evaluations N per M-lane and the maximum change rate σ for μ as well as a confidence window length L and an adaptation window length A. Set $k = 0$. Furthermore, select a learning threshold τ and the initial signal history length M_0. Set $M = M_0$, $W_{0,d} = \mathbf{e}_{\max(M+d,1)} \in \mathbb{R}^{\max(M+d,1)}$ for $d = -1,0,1$. d is used to describe the M-lanes.

2. Initialise $3N$ instances $\mathbf{P}_{\{1,-1\}}, \mathbf{P}_{\{1,0\}}, \mathbf{P}_{\{1,1\}}, \ldots, \mathbf{P}_{\{N,-1\}}, \mathbf{P}_{\{N,0\}}, \mathbf{P}_{\{N,1\}}$ of the prediction algorithm using

   - $\mu\left[\mathbf{P}_{\{i,d\}}\right] = \sigma\mu_k + 2(i-1)(\mu_k - \sigma\mu_k)/(N-1)$,
   - $M\left[\mathbf{P}_{\{i,d\}}\right] = \max(1, M+d)$,
   - $W\left[\mathbf{P}_{\{i,d\}}\right] = W_{k,d}$,

   for $i = 1,\ldots,N$ and $d = -1,0,1$. Here, $\{i,d\}$, the subscript of the $\mathbf{P}$'s, denotes the currently used lane: the first index, i, determines the μ-lane whereas the second index, d, determines the M-lane.
   Let $L_k = L$ and, as a notational shortcut, $\Lambda_k = L_0 + \cdots + L_{k-1}$.

3. Simultaneously evaluate the $3N$ algorithms and build $3N$ lists of predicted values. Allow the algorithms to perform up to sampling point $(k+1)A + \Lambda_k + L_k$. Use $\mathbf{P}_{\{\frac{N+1}{2},0\}}$ for the prediction on the window $[kA + \Lambda_k, (k+1)A + \Lambda_k + L_k]$.

4. Let $j(d)$, $d = -1,0,1$, be such that $\mathbf{P}_{\{j(d),d\}}$ is the predictor which has performed best out of the $\mathbf{P}_{\{i,d\}}$, $i = 1,\ldots,N$, on the last L sampling points. This means that $j(d)$ is the index of best μ-lane in the dth M-lane. Now let D be such that

$\mathbf{P}_{\{j(D),D\}}$ has performed best out of the $\mathbf{P}_{\{j(d),d\}}$, i.e., D is the index of the best of the three μ-lanes $j(-1)$ in the M-line -1, $j(0)$ in the M-line 0 and $j(1)$ in the M-line 1.

If the decrease in error between $\mathbf{P}_{\{j(D),D\}}$ and $\mathbf{P}_{\{\frac{N+1}{2},0\}}$ (the currently used predictor) is less than τ, increase L_k and go to step 3. Otherwise, set

- $M = \max(1, M+D)$,
- $W_{k+1,d} = W_{0,d} = \mathbf{e}_{\max(M+d,1)} \in \mathbb{R}^{\max(M+d,1)}$, $d = -1, 0, 1$,
- $\mu_{k+1} = \mu\left[\mathbf{P}_{\{j(D),D\}}\right]$.

Here, the new weights are preliminarily initialised to be unit vectors. This is done to discard possibly wrong weights if the new value of μ to be used for prediction is either $\sigma\mu_k$ or $(2-\sigma)\mu_k$. If this is not the case, i.e., if $\mu_{k+1} > \sigma\mu_k$ and $\mu_{k+1} < (2-\sigma)\mu_k$, we set $W_{k+1,d}$ to $W\left[\mathbf{P}_{\{j(d+D),d+D\}}\right]$ for those d where $-1 \leq d+D \leq 1$. This means that we use the weight vectors determined by the locally optimal predictor as initial weights for the next iteration as long as such vectors already exist.

5. Increase k and go to step 2.

Now the question of finding the optimal learning parameter μ and signal history length M has been reduced to selecting working parameters, i.e., values for which the algorithm does not diverge immediately. Furthermore, the selection of the lengths of the adaptation and confidence windows is not as crucial as long as the algorithms are given enough time to settle down prior to switching. Reasonable results can be obtained by setting the adaptation window to approximately ten and the confidence window to approximately five breathing cycles.

Example 9. We come back to example 8. To demonstrate the capabilities of the fast lane approach, the same signals were subjected to prediction with this method. The inital values for M and μ remained unchanged at 50 and 0.2, respectively. A was set to 1,000, L was set to 333, τ was set to 0.9, σ was set to 0.5 and N was set to 11. Applying the algorithms resulted in a reduction of RMS error to 0.057 (first signal) and 0.056 (second signal). Without the FLA, the errors were 0.13 on part 1, $2.19 \cdot 10^{10}$ on part 2a and 7.57 on part 2b. Since the signal was corrupted with Gaussian noise of 0.04 standard deviation, an RMS error of less than 0.06 comes very close to the theoretically obtainable value.

The FLA changed the values of μ and M only twice: on part 1, the values were changed to $\mu = 0.1$ and $M = 51$ at sample 1,126, on part 2a, the values were changed to $\mu = 0.05$ and $M = 52$ at sample 25,047 and on part 2b, the values were not changed, i.e., they remained at $\mu = 0.1$ and $M = 51$.

Example 10. In a second experiment, the error surface of the nLMS$_2$ algorithm (see example 5) for $p = 2$ was re-created using the FLA extension. The result is shown in figure 4.12. It is obvious that, although the optimal RMS value possible using the nLMS$_2$ algorithm is not reached, the FLA extension manages to produces better prediction in many cases. The parameters used for the FLA extension were $A \in \{150, 300, 600, 1000\}$, $T = A/3$, $\tau = 0.9$, $\sigma = 0.5$, $N = 11$.

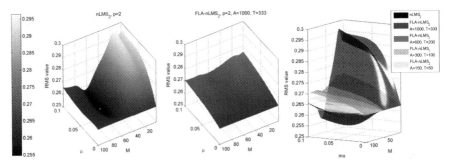

Fig. 4.12: RMS error plot of the nLMS$_2$ algorithm (left) and its FLA extension (centre) algorithm for $M = 1, \ldots, 100$ and $\mu \in [0, 0.1]$; evaluated on the real signal. It is clear that the FLA extension, although it does not reach the optimal value possible using the nLMS$_2$ algorithm, produces a much flatter surface. The right plot shows an overlay of the surfaces generated.

4.2.3 Multi-step Linear Methods (MULIN)

The basic idea of this new family of algorithms, first presented in [14, 15], is to compute the predicted signal from an expansion of the error signal, i.e., the difference of the measured signal y and the signal $D(y, \delta)$, which is the signal y delayed by δ samples. The simplest member of this family of prediction algorithms, MULIN0, is based on the following assumption:

Assumption 4.2 *Let y be the signal to predict and let δ be the prediction horizon. Then*

$$y_{k+\delta} - y_k \approx y_k - y_{k-\delta}.$$

Based on assumption 4.2, we define the simple linear prediction algorithm according to the following equation:

$$\hat{Y}_{k+\delta}^0 = y_k - \Delta(y, \delta)_k, \tag{4.22}$$

where $\Delta(y, \delta) = D(y, \delta) - y$.

Of course, this approach fails quite badly as soon as assumption 4.2 does not hold. This, obviously, is the case whenever the signal's first derivative changes. The next step is therefore to further expand the prediction error $\Delta(y, \delta)_k$ to take this change into account. This is done by taking higher order differences, i.e., by regarding the term $\Delta(y, \delta)_k$ in equation 4.22 as the unknown and to be predicted quantity. Applying equation 4.22 to $\Delta(y, \delta)_k$ results in the first-order prediction equation, shown in equation 4.23.

$$\hat{Y}_{k+\delta}^{1,M} = y_k - (\Delta(y, \delta)_k - \Delta(\Delta(y, \delta), M)_k)$$
$$= y_k - 2\Delta(y, \delta)_k + \Delta(y, \delta)_{k-M} \tag{4.23}$$

In this extended algorithm, a new parameter M was introduced. This parameter can be seen as something akin to the signal history length of LMS prediction algorithms: it controls how far back the algorithm should look to determine the change in the signal's first derivative. Naturally, we would expect M to be equal to δ since we are trying to predict the change of the difference signal $\Delta(y,\delta)$. In those cases, however, where the signal we try to predict is highly irregular or instable, either due to the presence of noise or high signal variation, or the sampling rate is low, it is reasonable to assume that the correlation between y_{k-M} and $y_{k+\delta}$ is higher the smaller M becomes. This is highlighted in figure 4.13. Nevertheless, when both the

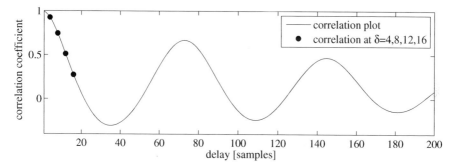

Fig. 4.13: Autocorrelation of a real breathing motion signal

sampling rate and the signal-to-noise ratio are high, we can assume that long-term signal dependencies exist. To exploit these dependencies, we repeat the expansion process, generating third and fourth order linear prediction algorithms. This is done by applying equation 4.22 to $\Delta(y,\delta)_k$, $\Delta(y,\delta)_{k-M}$ and $\Delta(y,\delta)_{k-2M}$.

$$\hat{Y}_{k+\delta}^{2,M} = y_k - 4\Delta(y,\delta)_k + 4\Delta(y,\delta)_{k-M} - \Delta(y,\delta)_{k-2M} \tag{4.24}$$

$$\hat{Y}_{k+\delta}^{3,M} = y_k - 8\Delta(y,\delta)_k + 12\Delta(y,\delta)_{k-M} - 6\Delta(y,\delta)_{k-2M} + \Delta(y,\delta)_{k-3M}$$

Clearly, in those cases where the correlation between the quantities $y_{k+\delta}$ and $\Delta(y,\delta)_{k-2M}$ as well as between $y_{k+\delta}$ and $\Delta(y,\delta)_{k-3M}$ is low, we do not expect improvement over the simple or first-order prediction algorithms, and, in fact, might even witness degradation of the prediction performance. This expansion process can now be repeated. The general expansion formula is given in theorem 1.

Theorem 1. *The preliminary MULIN algorithms given in equations 4.22 to 4.25 can be combined into*

$$\hat{Y}_{k+\delta}^{n,M} = y_k + \sum_{i=0}^{n} \left(\frac{(-1)^{i+1} 2^{n-i} n!}{i!(n-i)!} \Delta(y,\delta)_{k-iM} \right). \tag{4.25}$$

By repeating the expansion process, this formula also holds for higher order algorithms.

Proof. The theorem is proved by induction on n. For $n = 0$, we get

$$\hat{Y}_{k+\delta}^{0,M} = y_k + \frac{(-1)^{0+1}2^{0-0}0!}{0!(0-0)!}\Delta(y,\delta)_{k-0\cdot M} = y_k - \Delta(y,\delta)_k,$$

which is the formula given in equation 4.22. Now assume the formula to be correct up to n. We need to show that applying the expansion rule given in equation 4.22 to equation 4.25 gives the same result as replacing n by $n+1$ in equation 4.25, i.e.,

$$\sum_{i=0}^{n}\left(\frac{(-1)^{i+1}2^{n-i}n!}{i!(n-i)!}\left(2\Delta(y,\delta)_{k-iM} - \Delta(y,\delta)_{k-(i+1)M}\right)\right) =$$

$$= \sum_{i=0}^{n+1}\left(\frac{(-1)^{i+1}2^{n+1-i}(n+1)!}{i!(n+1-i)!}\Delta(y,\delta)_{k-iM}\right).$$

This is done by comparing coefficients of $\Delta(y,\delta)_{k-iM}$:

$\underline{\Delta(y,\delta)_k:}$

$$\frac{(-1)^{0+1}2^{n-0}n!}{0!(n-0)!}\cdot 2 = -2^{n+1} \qquad \frac{(-1)^{0+1}2^{n+1-0}(n+1)!}{0!(n+1-0)!} = -2^{n+1}$$

$\underline{\Delta(y,\delta)_{k-iM},\ i = 1,\ldots,n:}$

left:

$$\frac{(-1)^{i-1+1}2^{n-i+1}n!}{(i-1)!(n-i+1)!}\cdot(-1) + \frac{(-1)^{i+1}2^{n-i}n!}{i!(n-i)!}\cdot 2 =$$

$$= \frac{(-1)^{i+1}2^{n+1-i}n!}{(i-1)!(n+1-i)!} + \frac{(-1)^{i+1}2^{n+1-i}n!}{i!(n-i)!} =$$

$$= \frac{i(-1)^{i+1}2^{n+1-i}n! + (n+1-i)(-1)^{i+1}2^{n+1-i}n!}{i!(n+1-i)!} =$$

$$= \frac{(-1)^{i+1}2^{n+1-i}n!(n+1)}{i!(n+1-i)!} = \frac{(-1)^{i+1}2^{n+1-i}(n+1)!}{i!(n+1-i)!}$$

right:

$$\frac{(-1)^{i+1}2^{n+1-i}(n+1)!}{i!(n+1-i)!}$$

$\underline{\Delta(y,\delta)_{k-(n+1)M}:}$

$$\frac{(-1)^{n+1}2^{n-n}n!}{n!(n-n)!}(-1) = (-1)^{n+2} \qquad \frac{(-1)^{n+1+1}2^{n+1-n-1}(n+1)!}{(n+1)!(n+1-n-1)!} = (-1)^{n+2}$$

This completes the proof.

To exploit long-term dependencies, an exponential smoothing parameter $\mu \geq 0$ is introduced to form the final form of the MULIN algorithms, see equation 4.26.

$$\hat{y}_{k+\delta}^{\text{MULIN}n,M} = \mu \cdot \hat{Y}_{k+\delta}^{n,M} + (1-\mu) \cdot \hat{y}_{k+\delta-1}^{\text{MULIN}n,M}, \quad n \in \mathbb{N}_0 \qquad (4.26)$$

Example 11. Using the simulated and real respiratory motion data described in examples 4 and 5, the MULIN algorithms were evaluated for $n = 0, \ldots, 4$, $M = 1, \ldots, 100$ and $\mu \in [0,1]$. The error plots for the simulated signal are shown in figure 4.14, the plots for the real signal are shown in figure 4.15. Optimal parameters resulted in an RMS of 0.0361 (for $n = 1$, $M = 18$ and $\mu = 0.2943$) on the simulated signal and an RMS of 0.1687 (for $n = 2$, $M = 1$ and $\mu = 0.5195$) on the real signal.

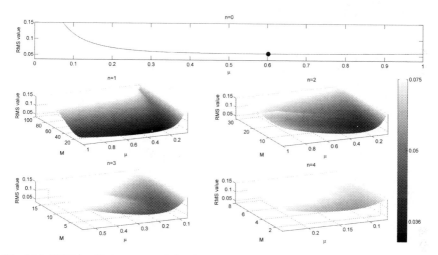

Fig. 4.14: **RMS prediction error of the different MULIN algorithms** ($n = 0,1,2,3,4$) **on the simulated signal from example 4. Degradation of prediction performance for $n \geq 2$ is clearly visible. Optimal performance of 0.0357 is obtained for $n = 1$, $M = 18$, $\mu = 0.2883$.**

4.2.4 Support Vector Regression

In recent works [17, 18], Support Vector Regression (SVR), an extension of the concept of Support Vector Machines (SVMs), has been used to predict respiratory motion for the first time. More details on the mathematical backround are given in section A.2.

To use SVR for respiratory motion prediction, we use training data

$$\left\{ (u_{k_1}, y_{k_1+\delta}), \ldots, (u_{k_L}, y_{k_L+\delta}) \right\}$$

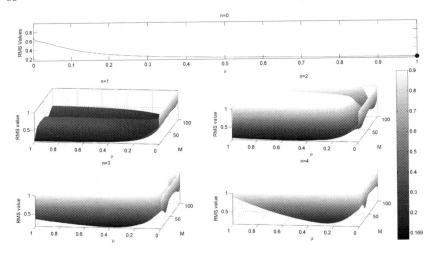

Fig. 4.15: RMS prediction error of the different MULIN algorithms ($n = 0, 1, 2, 3, 4$) on the real signal from example 5. Optimal performance of 0.1687 is obtained for $n = 2$, $M = 1$, $\mu = 0.5195$.

to find a function $f(x)$ that has at most ε deviation from the actually obtained targets $y_{i+\delta}$, i.e.,

$$|f(u_i) - y_{i+\delta}| \leq \varepsilon.$$

Here, u_i is some signal history vector from $\mathbb{R}^M$. The components of u_i are selected in some manner from the past part of the time series y, i.e., $u_{i,j} = y_{g(i,j)}$ where g is strictly monotonously decreasing in i, $g(i, 1) = i$ and $g(i, j) \geq 1$ for all j.

Prediction of Human Respiratory Motion

Up to now, prediction of human respiratory motion using kernel-based machine learning methods has not been investigated much. One reason is that, until very recently, prediction with support vector regression required either constant re-training of the SVR function or the assumption of stationarity. With [27], however, it has become possible to implement support vector regression for online prediction by iteratively forgetting older samples and adding new measurements to the SVR function without having to completely re-train it. Some problems remain, however:

1. Choice of kernel function and corresponding parameters
2. Selection of the SVR parameters C, the penalty factor, and ε, the error insensitivity level
3. Selection of the signal history to avoid the curse of dimensionality [39]
4. Computational time is still very high and might prohibit real-time applications

The proposed prediction algorithm, called Support Vector Regression prediction (SVRpred), was implemented in C++ using the Accurate Online Support Vector

Regression (AOSVR) library created by Francesco Parella [29]. Available kernel functions are:

- linear, i.e., $k(x,y) = \langle x,y \rangle$,
- polynomial, i.e., $k(x,y) = (\sigma \langle x,y \rangle + \tau)^n$,
- Gaussian Radial Basis Function (RBF), i.e., $k(x,y) = \exp\left(-\frac{\|x-y\|_2^2}{2\sigma^2}\right)$,
- Exponential RBF, i.e., $k(x,y) = \exp\left(-\frac{\|x-y\|_1^2}{2\sigma^2}\right)$
- Hyperbolic tangent, i.e., $k(x,y) = \tanh\left(\sigma \langle x,y \rangle + \tau\right)$

Selecting the Signal History

Since the proposed prediction method is based on regression, we need to select a subset of previous samples to use as input vector for the SVR machine. Naturally, one would start with selecting a signal history length M, ideally a multiple of the prediction horizon δ, and take all old samples between t_n, the current position in time, and t_{n-M+1} to try to predict $t_{n+\delta}$ from these. In our application, however, when we deal with high-frequency sampling, we may have a prediction horizon of up to 200 samples (see [25]) and thus end up trying to model an extremely high dimensional signal even when using moderate signal history lengths of 2δ, say.

Furthermore, it seems reasonable to assume that the intrinsic dimension of the regressor of dimension M is probably less than M. Unfortunately, we cannot employ the tools proposed in [39] to reduce the dimensionality of the regressor (like Principal Component Analysis (PCA), Curvilinear Component Analysis [5], Curvilinear Distance Analysis [26] and Isomaps [37]) since the sensory input data available changes as time progresses and we might thus face a change of intrinsic dimension when breathing patterns change. We therefore decided to take a more conventional approach: to reduce the dimension of the regressor by simply skipping input samples. Therefore the signal history is either linearly or quadratically spread out, i.e., we do not take the samples at

$$t_n, t_{n-1}, t_{n-2}, \ldots, t_{n-M+1}$$

but instead we take either the samples at

$$t_n, t_{n-l}, t_{n-2l}, \ldots, t_{n-(M-1)l}$$

or at

$$t_n, t_{n-l^2}, t_{n-(2l)^2}, t_{n-(3l)^2}, \ldots, t_{n-((M-1)l)^2},$$

where l is called the stepping parameter.

Prediction method

Using these simplifications, the initial version of the proposed prediction method is outlined below:

For each sample n,

1. build the signal history

$$u_n = \left(y_n, y_{n-l^a}, y_{n-(2l)^a}, y_{n-(3l)^a}, \ldots, y_{n-((M-1)l)^a} \right)^{\mathrm{T}},$$

2. update the SVR machine, i.e., train the sample pair $\{u_{n-\delta}, y_n\}$,
3. compute the prediction value $\hat{y}_{n+\delta}$ from u_n using the SVR prediction formula (see equation A.14),
4. if more than R training sample pairs are used in the SVR machine, remove the oldest one, i.e., retrain the machine without the sample pair $\{u_{n-\delta-R+1}, y_{n-R+1}\}$.

Here, $a \in \{1, 2\}$ and $l \in \mathbb{N}$ are parameters controlling the step size (i.e., linear or quadratic spacing) and $R \in \mathbb{N}$ determines the minimum number of samples required in the machine's memory.

A pseudo-code listing of this algorithm can be found in listing E.1.

Optimisation for Speed

One drawback of the SVRpred method is that on today's business PCs computational speed is not high enough. To evaluate and possibly alleviate this problem, we propose to train and forget only a subset of all samples instead of training each new measurement and subsequently forgetting the oldest sample. Steps two and four of the above process are changed as follows after introducing the training percentage τ:

2a. if $n \equiv 0 \bmod \lfloor 1/\tau \rfloor$, update the SVR machine by training the sample pair $\{u_{n-\delta}, y_n\}$
4a. if $n \equiv 0 \bmod \lfloor 1/\tau \rfloor$ and if more than τR training sample pairs are used in the SVR machine, remove the oldest one, i.e., re-train the machine without the sample pair $\{u_{n-\delta-\tau R+1}, y_{n-\tau R+1}\}$

A pseudo-code listing of this algorithm can be found in listing E.2.

Parameter Selection

As mentioned before, the selection of the parameters of the SVRpred algorithm may be very difficult. Especially selecting the training insensitivity level ε and the signal history length M (and the stepping parameter l) are not straight-forward. Since the optimal values for these parameters—as well as for C, τ and the kernel's parameters—cannot be determined in the setting of online prediction, we propose to select these values as follows:

- ε should be set to the standard deviation of the noise present in the signal. On a simulated signal, this value is known and can be used directly. On a real signal, however, this value is unknown. It is possible to resort to approximating this value using the aforementiond wavelet smoothing method (see section 3.3):

$$\varepsilon \approx \mathrm{std}\left((W_{1,1},\ldots,W_{1,N})^{\mathsf{T}}\right)$$

Here, W_1 is the first scale of the à trous wavelet decomposition of the signal y.
- M can be selected by looking at the correlation coefficients of the signal and its lags. Let $x_m = \Delta(y, m+\delta)$. We then can compute

$$\chi_m = \frac{\sum_{i=1}^{N-\delta-m}(x_{m,i}-\bar{x}_m)(y_i-\bar{y})}{\sqrt{\sum_{i=1}^{N-\delta-m}(x_{m,i}-\bar{x}_m)^2 \sum_{i=1}^{N-\delta-m}(y_i-\bar{y})^2}},$$

i.e., the autocorrelation coefficient for different lags $m = 1,\ldots,200$. Here, $\bar{x}_m$ and $\bar{y}$ denote the mean values of x_m and y, respectively. Then M can be selected such that $\chi_m \geq 0.6$ for all $m = 1,\ldots,M$.

To determine M and ε, only the first couple of breathing cycles of a signal should be used and these samples should subsequently be disregarded when computing the prediction error.

Setting proper values for C and the kernel parameters as well as the training share τ, however, cannot be done in this way. The following example will give insight into determining the influence of these values.

Example 12. Consider the real respiratory motion signal that was presented in example 5. To determine the importance of the SVR penalty term C, the kernel parameters, and the training percentage τ, two experiments were performed. First, the relative RMS error of the SVRpred algorithm was computed for multiple values of C and σ (in all experiments, the Gaussian RBF kernel function is used) using optimal values of ε and M, which were selected using a grid search. Second, the values of M and ε were set according to the above ideas, resulting in $M = 5$ and $\varepsilon = 0.0355$ and the SVRpred algorithm was evaluated using $C = 20$ and $\sigma = 2$ for varying values of τ. The results of both experiments are shown in figure 4.16. What is clear is that the selection of C does not have much influence on the prediction result, whereas the selection of σ is somewhat relevant (figure 4.16a). Additionally, it is obvious that an increase in τ results in a decrease of RMS and simultaneous increase in prediction time (figure 4.16b). In all experiments, R was set to 2,000.

We can thus deduce that, for the sample signal presented, we can safely select $C = 30$, $\sigma = 2$ and $\tau = 0.1$. To validate the parameter selection ideas for ε and M, another example is provided.

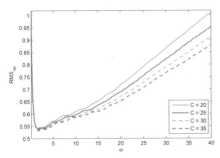

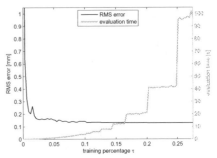

(a) For each pair (C,σ), the optimal values for ε and M were determined and the resulting relative RMS is shown. $l = 1$, $\tau = 0.1$.

(b) Evaluation of the impact of training percentage τ on relative RMS (black) and evaluation time (grey). $\varepsilon = 0.0355$, $M = 5$, $l = 1$, $C = 30$, $\sigma = 2$.

Fig. 4.16: Evaluation of the SVRpred algorithm on real data for different values of C and σ, subfigure (a), as well as for different values of τ, subfigure (b).

Example 13. With the same signal as before and using $C = 20$, $\sigma = 2$, $\tau = 0.1$, prediction performance was evaluated for changing values of ε and M. ε ranged from 0 to 0.3 and M from 1 to 60. The evaluation results are shown in figure 4.17. We found that the optimal RMS error of 0.1431 was obtained for $\varepsilon = 0.0061$ and $M = 5$, reasonably close to the predicted values of $\varepsilon = 0.0355$ and $M = 5$. Had we used these values, the RMS error would have been 0.1446, a difference of merely 1.01 %. In terms of relative RMS, this amounts to a difference of 0.586 percentage points.

What we can also see, however, is that minimal RMS does not necessarily coincide with minimal jitter: using the optimal values for ε and M, the jitter $\mathfrak{J}$ was found to be $1.930\frac{mm}{s}$, nowhere near the lowest obtainable value of $1.185\frac{mm}{s}$. Note that the original signal's jitter is $1.416\frac{mm}{s}$. Clearly, the dilemma postulated in section 3.2, that optimality of different error measures do not necessarily coincide, is indeed true.

Third, the evaluation time of the algorithm was determined to be 4.42 s. This corresponds to an average prediction time per sample of 0.57 ms, well under the theoretical limit of 38.5 ms (corresponding to the sampling rate of 26 Hz). This shows that the SVRpred algorithm—using moderate values of τ and M—is suitable for real-time applications despite its relatively high computational complexity.

4.3 Predicting Smoothed Signals[3]

The signals from the moving target study of section 3.4 were also subjected to prediction to test the applicability of the wavelet-based smoothing method (see sec-

---

[3] Parts of this section have been published in [12]

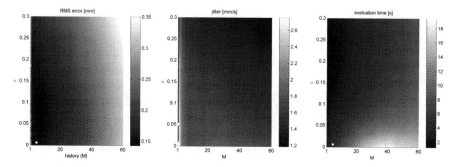

Fig. 4.17: Evaluation results of the SVRpred algorithm for different values of ε and M. The left panel shows the resulting RMS error, the centre panel shows the resulting jitter $\mathfrak{J}$ and the right panel shows the prediction time needed. The point corresponding to optimal RMS is marked with a circle. Optimal RMS of 0.1431 mm was achieved for $\varepsilon = 0.0061$ and $M = 5$, corresponding to a jitter $\mathfrak{J}$ of 1.930 $\frac{mm}{s}$ and an evaluation time of 4.42 s.

tion 3.3) to clinical settings. We applied the nLMS$_2$ algorithm (see section 4.2.1.1) and the MULIN family of algorithms (see section 4.2.3) to the signal obtained using system (F) in experiments with a robotic system (see section 3.4.1.2) and with a volunteer in our lab (see section 3.4.1.3). The prediction horizon considered was 150 ms. Prediction was done using the graphical toolkit developed at our lab, see section 4.4. The prediction algorithms' parameters were optimised using a grid search such as to minimise the residual RMS error, disregarding the value of $\mathfrak{J}$. For the synthetic signal, we can see that even moderate smoothing results in a tremendous improvement of signal stability: the jitter of the predicted signal drops by up to 95 %, depending on the algorithm employed (figure 4.19a, bottom row). Similarly, the prediction error drops by up to 37 % for the nLMS$_2$ algorithm but hardly changes for the MULIN family of algorithms (figure 4.19a, top row). In these figures, we use the notion of relative RMS and jitter, which are computed according to definitions 2, 9, 10 and 11.

It is clear that smoothing eventually starts to degrade prediction performance since the additional delay incurred by the smoothing algorithm (see section 3.3) needs to be compensated. Therefore the level of smoothing needs to be carefully determined: it is a trade-off between reduction of jitter and possible increase of prediction error. Analysis of the real respiratory motion signal recorded in section 3.4 reveals that it has an average respiratory frequency of 0.35 Hz with a standard deviation of 0.1 Hz. This shows that it conforms well to the limits of typical respiraton described in section 3.3. Figure 4.18 shows the spectra of both the original signal (black) and the smoothed signal $\mathscr{W}_4(y)$ (grey). It is clear that high frequencies are strongly attenuated and that the main frequencies—i.e., the frequencies corresponding to respiratory motion—remain largely the same (see the inset). We can thus use the signal $\mathscr{W}_4(y)$ as reference signal for further evaluation.

Again, application of wavelet smoothing does lead to a decrease in prediction error, albeit not as significant as with the synthetic signals. However, the jitter of the predicted signals drops strongly—by as much as 95 % (see figure 4.19b, bottom). For

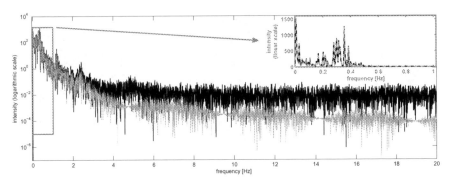

Fig. 4.18: Spectra of the breathing signal from figure 3.16 (black) and of the smoothed signal (grey; scales 1 to 4 discarded). Note the logarithmic scale in the intensity. The inset shows an enlargement of the frequency range from 0 to 1 Hz (linear scale of intensity). Here we can clearly see that the smoothed signal and the original signal coincide very well.

the $nLMS_2$ algorithm, the prediction error drops by up to 30 % (see figure 4.19b, top) while the MULIN algorithms seem to be relatively robust against noise and thus do not profit from smoothing. Again, the trade-off between reduction of jitter and better prediction becomes obvious, most notably so in the z-component of the motion signal where smoothing hardly influences prediction accuracy. An overview of all results is given in table 4.2. Note that here, the values of n and K were selected such as to get the best possible prediction (i.e., lowest RMS) while accepting possibly sub-optimal results for $\mathfrak{J}$. The optimisation—the same process as in generating figure 4.19b—was a simple evaluation of the prediction algorithms for all possible combinations of n, K and the algorithms' own parameters.

When predicting the real respiratory motion signal recorded in our lab, we only used the signal recorded using system (F). The reason for this is that it was the only system available to us for which we could readily manufacture the mentioned LED net and were able to track each LED individually. Furthermore, using one of the other systems—all of which operate at a much lower sampling frequency—the positive effects of smoothing will be lost. This is due to the fact that with lower tracking frequencies the effect of temporal delay added by smoothing (see equation 3.2) becomes more important. For a signal sampled at 60 Hz, the prediction horizon of 150 ms corresponds to 9 samples. Consequently, an additional seven samples from smoothing at level four ($\delta_4 = 7$) will result in an effective prediction horizon of approximately 267 ms. Applying the same level of smoothing when using the net with system (F) results in an effective prediction horizon of approximately 200 ms. This shows that, in clinical practice, it is important to move towards higher-frequency tracking to allow for effective pre-processing of the signal.

Another important question is how smoothing could be brought to clinical practice. As outlined in section 3.3 and section 4.3, we propose to construct a reference signal for real motion from the actually measured motion: this could be done in the clinic by recording 1-2 minutes of motion and determining the average breathing frequency. By selecting a cut-off frequency sufficiently far from this frequency (i.e.,

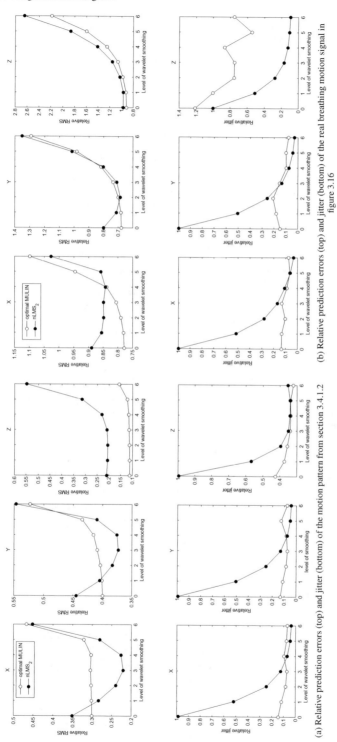

(a) Relative prediction errors (top) and jitter (bottom) of the motion pattern from section 3.4.1.2

(b) Relative prediction errors (top) and jitter (bottom) of the real breathing motion signal in figure 3.16

Fig. 4.19: Effect of smoothing on prediction RMS and jitter

Table 4.2: Changes in prediction accuracy. K and n are the optimal values for the level of smoothing and the level of the MULIN algorithms, respectively.

(a) simulated data

		MULIN$_n$			nLMS$_2$	
no smoothing						
coord.	n	RMS$_{rel}$	J_{rel}		RMS$_{rel}$	J_{rel}
x	0	30.01	14.50		35.13	98.76
y	0	39.95	13.16		44.46	99.41
z	0	11.14	42.60		20.87	99.58
with smoothing						
coord.	K n	RMS$_{rel}$	J_{rel}	K	RMS$_{rel}$	J_{rel}
x	0 0	30.01	14.50	3	22.03	12.51
y	0 0	39.95	13.16	3	37.26	13.21
z	0 0	11.14	42.60	2	20.51	39.59

(b) real data

		MULIN$_n$			nLMS$_2$	
no smoothing						
coord.	n	RMS$_{rel}$	J_{rel}		RMS$_{rel}$	J_{rel}
x	2	77.82	13.45		100.00	99.95
y	1	67.81	14.20		100.00	99.95
z	2	91.65	121.10		100.00	99.96
with smoothing						
coord.	K n	RMS$_{rel}$	J_{rel}	K	RMS$_{rel}$	J_{rel}
x	0 2	77.82	13.45	4	84.26	10.85
y	0 1	67.81	14.20	3	68.60	13.51
z	0 2	91.65	121.10	1	96.97	51.19

10-20 times higher), we can be sure that—as detailed in the spectral analysis of the motion trace—no relevant information about respiratory motion is lost. With this constructed reference signal, it will then be possible to determine—also prior to treatment—which smoothing level yields the best prediction performance both in terms of RMS and jitter.

4.4 Graphical Prediction Toolkit[4]

To be able to easily analyse, evaluate, and demonstrate different prediction algorithms, a prediction toolkit has been developed. This tool allows the user to manipulate the input data, the algorithms' parameters and perform predictions and evaluations. To be more flexible, three modes of interaction with the toolkit are possible:

- Direct inclusion in own programmes as a library

---

[4] Parts of this section have been published in [34]

- CLI to use it as a stand alone evaluation tool
- GUI for intuitive use

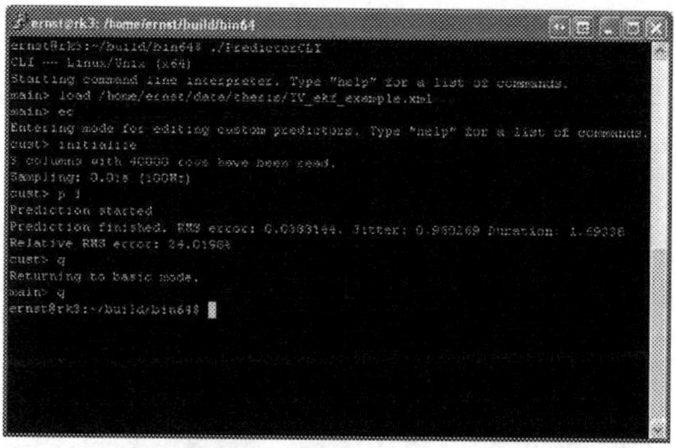

Fig. 4.20: The CLI toolkit running on Debian Linux (Squeeze, x64)

To allow maximum flexibility, the toolkit was implemented separated into three parts: a core library handling actual prediction and data input/output, a controller class providing high level features like loading and saving configurations, optimisation and evaluation, and the graphical and command line frontends. Two other design objectives were modularity and portability. Since not every user may require all prediction algorithms and other researchers may wish to contribute algorithms without having to deal with the implementation of the core library, the controller or the front-end, the algorithms were encapsulated into dynamically loadable files (DLLs on Windows, shared objects on Linux/Unix). Additionally, an Extensible Markup Language (XML) file describing the algorithm must accompany the library. These files describe the parameters available to the front-end, the parameters' default values, their possible ranges and can also contain detailed explanation about each parameter or the algorithm in general. The graphical front-end thus creates a dynamic interface for each loaded prediction library, displaying the parameters described in the XML file. Figure 4.20 shows a screen shot of the CLI toolkit running on Debian Linux (Squeeze, x64). Figure 4.21 shows the GUI running on Windows XP.

To allow maximum portability, the core library, the controller class and the command line front-end were written in ISO C++. It should be possible to compile the code on most systems. This is achieved by using the CMake cross-platform build tools [4], which dynamically generate the proper project files for a multitude of C/C++ compilers. We have successsfully compiled and tested the system on Windows xp/Vista/7 (32bit and 64bit), ubuntu, Debian and CentOS Linux (32bit and 64bit), MacOS X, and Sun Solaris 9 (running on SPARC). Implementation of the graphical front end was done using ISO C++ and the wxWidgets library [41]. The GUI has been successfully used on Windows xp/Vista/7 (32bit and 64bit), ubuntu,

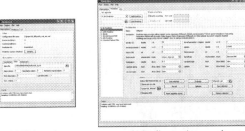

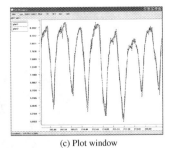

(a) Main options   (b) Predicor options panel   (c) Plot window
panel

Fig. 4.21: The GUI toolkit running on Windows xp

Debian and CentOS Linux (32bit and 64bit) and MacOS X. An overview of supported and tested platforms is given in table 4.3.

Table 4.3: Operating systems and architectures supported by PredictorGUI and Predictor-CLI. Entries marked with ✓have been tested, entries marked with (✓) should work and entries marked with — are untested.

	PredictorCLI	PredictorGUI
Windows xp/Vista/7 (i386 & x64)	✓	✓
ubuntu, Debian, CentOS Linux (i386 & x64)	✓	✓
other Linux	(✓)	(✓)
MacOS X (i386)	✓	✓
Solaris 9 (SPARC)	✓	— (a)

(a) We did not have access to the wxWidgets library on Solaris 9 (SPARC).

In general, the toolkit provides the following functions, both via the CLI and the GUI:

- Simple optimisation of algorithmic parameters by means of a grid search (built-in)
- Optimisation of algorithmic parameters using the active set algorithm presented in [21] (makes use of the ALGLIB library [1])
- Evaluation of an algorithm using ranges of parameters, including the support of multiple CPUs or cores for parallel evaluation
- Generation of output of the evaluation process readable by MATLAB®
- Simple plotting tools to display the predicted signal
- Wavelet-based preprocessing of the input data [9, 12] as outlined in section 3.3
- Simple batch processing and a command line interpreter (sample code is shown in listing E.4 in appendix E)
- Exporting of configurations for easy reproducability

- Master-slave system to allow distributed computing on multiple machines

At the moment, the following algorithms are supported by the toolkit:

- MULIN (external library)
- Multi-frequency based EKF tracking (external library)
- wLMS (external library)
- RLS (external library)
- SVRpred (external library)
- LMS, nLMS and their FLA extensions (built-in)
- no prediction (built-in)

Integration of other algorithms into the toolkit is easily possible by using the described framework.

4.5 Evaluating the Prediction Algorithms

Throughout this chapter, two signals have been used repeatedly for demonstrating the prediction algorithms' capabilities and shortcomings: a computer-generated signal simulating respiration (introduced in example 4), and a real-world respiratory motion trace recorded during a CyberKnife treatment session[5]. Before delving deeper into comparing the prediction results of the algorithms introduced in this work, the optimal prediction results on these two signals, which were, for the most part, acquired in the examples of this chapter, are summarised in table 4.4.

Table 4.4: Summary of the prediction results on a simulated and a real motion signal, optimal values are in bold

algorithm	simulated signal RMS (RMS_{rel})	jitter $\mathfrak{J}$	time[a]	real signal RMS (RMS_{rel})	jitter $\mathfrak{J}$	time[a]
no pred.	0.162 (100.00)	1.892	—	0.262 (100.00)	1.416	—
EKF	0.038 (23.36)	**1.008**	0.842	0.192 (73.30)	1.937	1.122
nLMS	0.040 (24.86)	2.219	0.475	0.200 (76.32)	**1.879**	0.011
RLS	**0.032** (**19.75**)	1.198	1.134	0.158 (60.43)	2.905	0.002
wLMS	0.046 (28.21)	1.911	1.821	0.149 (56.99)	2.114	0.927
MULIN	0.036 (22.09)	1.676	**0.007**	0.169 (64.36)	2.642	**0.001**
SVRpred	0.032 (20.04)	2.149	63.840	**0.143** (**55.16**)	1.930	2.470

[a] All timings were determined using Windows xp x64 Edition, running on a machine with an Intel® Core™ i7 940 CPU and 12 GiB of RAM. Evaluation was performed using one core only, the algorithms are not parallelised.

This data shows us that, even in this simple case, no algorithm is optimal from all points of view. In terms of RMS error, the SVRpred algorithm is best on the real-

---

[5] data by courtesy of Dr. Sonja Dieterich, Stanford University Cancer Center

world signal but it is outperformed by the RLS algorithm ever so slightly on the simulated signal.

4.5.1 A Respiratory Motion Database

To get a better feel for the quality of the different prediction algorithms, they have been evaluated on a large database of respiratory motion traces. The database consists of 304 motion traces recorded during CyberKnife treatment of 31 patients. The patients were treated with up to seven fractions, a total of 102 fractions were delivered. During each fraction, three markers were recorded. Markers two and three of one fraction were defect. The datasets range in duration from 80 to 158 minutes. The data was acquired at a frequency of approximately 26 Hz.

Data processing

Since the data was recorded during regular treatment, the data sets do not only show respiratory motion, but also the motion of the treatment couch whenever the patient was aligned or re-aligned. This can be seen in figure 4.22a: there are multiple couch movements prior to a longer period of relatively constant respiration. Only the longest period without couch motion was used for evaluation. In this sample case, the portion used is marked with a black rectangle and enlarged. Additionally, since respiratory motion predominantly occurs perpendicular to the chest wall, the data was reduced to its principle component. Figure 4.22b shows an enlargement of the area marked with the dotted rectangle in figure 4.22a after applying PCA. After processing, the signals had a length between 6.5 and 132 minutes, with an average of 71 minutes.

4.5.2 Comparing the Algorithms

To compare the results of the prediction algorithms, they were evaluated using the presented prediction toolkit (see section 4.4). The prediction horizon was set to four samples, corresponding to a latency of approximately 150 ms, well in line with the latency of the CyberKnife. The learning window was set to 2,000 samples, i.e., the prediction result on this part was not used for determining the RMS error. Consequently, this is the range of data used for frequency determination of the EKF algorithm, the value R of the SVRpred algorithm and the range of data on which the wLMS algorithm determines the regression depths a_j. To speed up parameter optimisation, the workload was distributed to seven machines in our department's laboratory running different versions and flavours of ubuntu (8.04, 8.10, 9.04, 10.04; i386 and x64) and Debian (Lenny x64) Linux with two to eight cores and frequen-

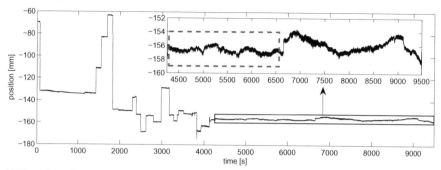

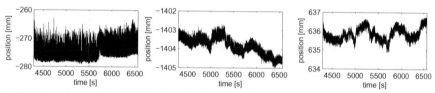

(a) The main graph shows the x-coordinate of the signal. We can clearly see large, sudden movements (due to couch repositioning) on top of the respiratory motion pattern. The data used for algorithm evaluation is marked with a black rectangle, enlarged at top right. The data marked with a dotted rectangle is subject to PCA and shown in figure 4.22b.

(b) The three motion directions of the signal marked with a dotted rectangle and shown in figure 4.22a. The motion range of the three components is 16.05, 2.26, and 1.88 mm, respectively.

Fig. 4.22: Sample trajectory of the respiratory motion data base (patient ID 20, fraction ID 71, marker ID 2).

cies ranging from 1.8 to 3.4 GHz. This makes comparison of evaluation times impossible.

Determining optimal parameters

To determine the theoretically optimal RMS errors of the prediction algorithms, optimisation of the algorithmic parameters was performed. Four different approaches were taken:

1. Exhaustive grid search evaluation covering the complete range of parameters
2. A bound constrained optimisation method suitable for nonlinear functions
3. Reduced grid search around parameters determined optimal for one signal
4. Using parameters optimal for one signal for prediction on all signals

Clearly, to determine the best possible results, an exhaustive grid search is ideal: using this approach, local minima can be avoided and the result is guaranteed to be optimal. This method, however, can only be used if both the algorithm's run time is short and the number and range of parameters is limited. Consequently, it was only used for the MULIN and nLMS algorithms. A typical evaluation run consisted of 5,000 (nLMS) to 100,000 (MULIN) function evaluations.

The second-best approach then is to use an optimisation method. While such methods are not guaranteed to find the global minimum, they will usually converge to a
local minimum. We have used the active set bounded optimisation routine outlined
in [21], which is implemented in the open-source ALGLIB library [1]. To be able to
use this algorithm, numeric differentiation of the algorithms' RMS error with respect to the parameters was implemented, using a five-point stencil where possible.
This requirement already shows that the optimisation method will require a substan-
tial number of function evaluations and, on top, requires the RMS error surface to
be smooth. We have used this approach for optimisation of the RLS algorithm's parameters. It was not possible to use it for the EKF algorithm, since this algorithm's
error surface is very noisy (see figure 4.2). The SVRpred algorithm was also optimised using this approach, although the ranges of its parameters were restricted
beforehand.

The third approach, the reduced grid search method, was used for the EKF method.
Since it is possible to restrict the parameters' ranges, the amount of evaluations
needed per signal could be reduced greatly. Here, a typical evaluation run consisted
of 100 to 1,000 function evaluations.

For the wLMS method, even 100 to 1,000 evaluations would take too much time:
evaluating these algorithms for one set of parameters may require up to three minutes (on a machine with an Intel Core i7 940 CPU, 12 GiB RAM, running ubuntu
9.10 x64). To reduce the work load, optimal parameters for one signal were determined and the algorithm was evaluated on the other signals using the same set of
parameters.

Results

After evaluating all algorithms on all 304 test signals, we see that, in terms of RMS
error, the nLMS algorithm is the algorithm performing worst, the EKF algorithm is
only slightly better, the RLS algorithm comes next and the MULIN, SVRpred and
wLMS algorithms perform similarly with an advantage for the wLMS algorithm.
When we look at the jitter of the predicted signals, however, the picture changes:
here, the EKF and nLMS algorithms perform very good: in most cases, the predicted
signals' jitter is only slightly larger than the original jitter. The SVRpred algorithm's
jitter is only marginally larger, whereas the wLMS algorithm has a noticeably higher
jitter, the MULIN algorithm's jitter is even higher still and the RLS algorithm may
produce a jitter as much as four times the original jitter. These findings are illustrated in figure 4.23. If we look at how often each individual algorithm provided the
lowest RMS (or jitter), these findings are confirmed: the wLMS algorithm performs
best in more than 60 % of the cases, the SVRpred algorithm in 30 % of the cases, the
MULIN algorithm in another 5.9 %, whereas the nLMS and RLS algorithms both
result in the lowest RMS error in only 1.6 % of cases. The EKF algorithm is never
the best algorithm. Again, the picture changes somewhat when looking at the jitter:
here, the EKF algorithm is best in 38 % of the cases, followed by the nLMS algorithm with 31 % and the SVRpred algorithm with 24 % of the cases. The MULIN

algorithm is optimal in only 4.6 % of the cases and the RLS algorithm in 1.6 %. The wLMS algorithm never produces the lowest jitter. These numbers are given in table 4.5.

It is very interesting to see that, although the other algorithms were at least partially optimised, the wLMS algorithm—which used the same parameters for all signals—did so much better in terms of RMS error.

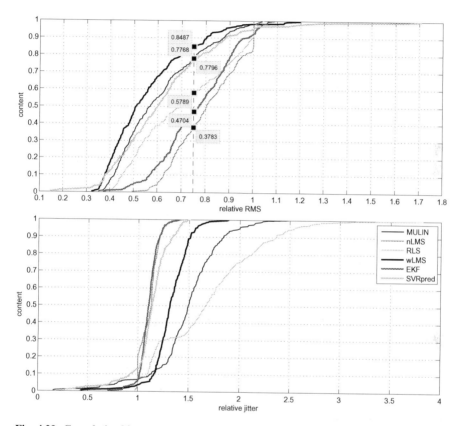

Fig. 4.23: **Cumulative histogram of the prediction performance on the respiratory motion database. The top panel shows the relative RMS obtained, the bottom panel shows the relative jitter. Read: a relative RMS error of at most 0.75 was obtained in 38 % of the cases using the nLMS algorithm, in 47 % of the cases using the EKF algorithm, in 58 % of the cases using the RLS algorithm, in 78 % of the cases using the MULIN or SVRpred algorithms, and in 85 % of the cases using the wLMS algorithm.**

We now turn to see how far away from the minimal RMS obtained using the best algorithm the other algorithms are. In the case of the MULIN and wLMS algorithms, we see that the difference in relative RMS to the optimal algorithm is below 0.16 in 90 % of the cases. This figure increases to 0.29 for the SVRpred, to 0.33 for the RLS, to 0.39 for the EKF, and to 0.42 for the nLMS algorithms. The complete

Table 4.5: Amount of optimal results delivered by each individual algorithm (one signal corresponds to 0.33 %)

	MULIN	nLMS	RLS	wLMS	EKF	SVRpred
relative RMS	5.92 %	1.64 %	1.64 %	60.86 %	—	29.93 %
relative jitter	4.61 %	31.25 %	1.64 %	—	38.16 %	24.34 %

histograms and cumulative histograms of these differences are shown in figure 4.24 and figure 4.25.

When we look at the statistics of these differences, we can see that always using the wLMS, MULIN or SVRpred algorithms will, most of the time, only result in a relative RMS which is about 0.1 larger than the best possible value. The numbers are given in table 4.6.

Table 4.6: Statistical values of the differences in relative RMS between the optimal values and the values obtained by the individual algorithms

	MULIN	nLMS	RLS	wLMS	EKF	SVRpred
mean value	0.0763	0.2781	0.1760	0.0613	0.2315	0.1319
median value	0.0554	0.2682	0.1512	0.0372	0.2181	0.0923
maximal value	0.6219	0.8342	0.8479	0.5333	0.8408	0.7900
standard deviation	0.0745	0.1215	0.1202	0.0861	0.1195	0.1336

We now focus on the three algorithms performing best, the MULIN, wLMS and SVRpred methods. It is interesting to see that the prediction errors of these methods are strongly correlated. Figure 4.26 shows a 3D plot where each dot corresponds to the evaluation of the three algorithms on one signal. The x-axis shows the error of the MULIN algorithm, the y-axis the error of the wLMS algorithm, and the z-axis the error of the SVRpred algorithm. In the plot, the grey box encloses those signals for which all three algorithms resulted in an RMS_{rel} of less than 0.9. The corresponding signals are shown with circles. The open squares correspond to signals for which at least one algorithm resulted in an RMS_{rel} of more than 0.9. As mentioned before, the correlation between the errors is strong: the correlation coefficients are 0.95 (MULIN to wLMS), 0.76 (wLMS to SVRpred), and 0.68 (MULIN to SVRpred). This becomes clearer in figure 4.27, which shows the three 2D projections of figure 4.26. In both figures, five signals are marked with open circles: the best and worst signal for both the MULIN and SVRpred algorithms and one signal with medium values for all algorithms. These signals will be investigated further, their RMS prediction errors are listed in table 4.7.

Looking closer at these signals reveals that both S1 and S3 are very regular, with high average amplitude and Signal to noise ratio (SNR). S2 and S4, however, are very irregular: their amplitudes vary considerably, there is more noise and the si-

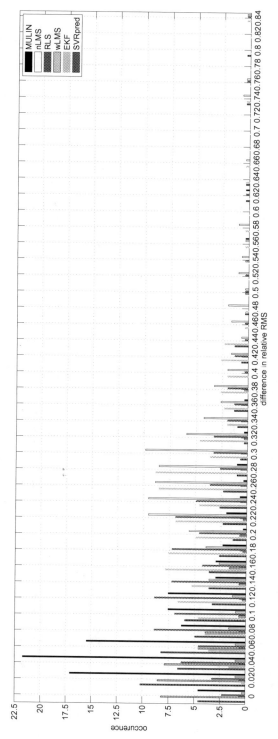

Fig. 4.24: Histogram of the differences between each algorithm's relative RMS values and the optimal RMS value. For each algorithm, only those signals were selected where the algorithm did not perform best.

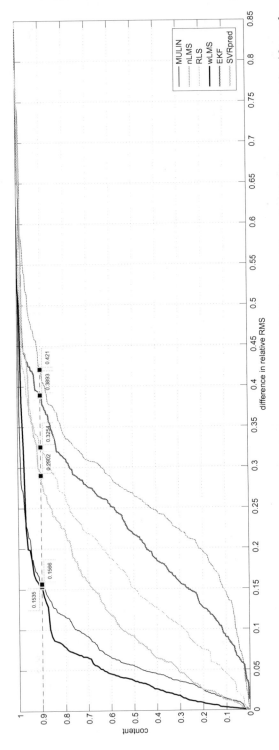

Fig. 4.25: Cumulative histogram of the differences between each algorithm's relative RMS values and the optimal RMS value. For each algorithm, only those signals were selected where the algorithm did not perform best.

Table 4.7: RMS errors of the five signals marked with circles in figure 4.26

signal	ID	description	MULIN	wLMS	SVRpred
S1	P34_F96_M2	best MULIN	35.22 %	33.18 %	32.77 %
S2	P43_F119_M2	worst MULIN	103.47 %	113.03 %	116.19 %
S3	P15_F53_M2	best SVRpred	42.50 %	37.16 %	14.58 %
S4	P32_F93_M1	worst SVRpred	96.04 %	98.71 %	171.00 %
S5	P20_F73_M2	medium values	82.05 %	81.86 %	87.81 %

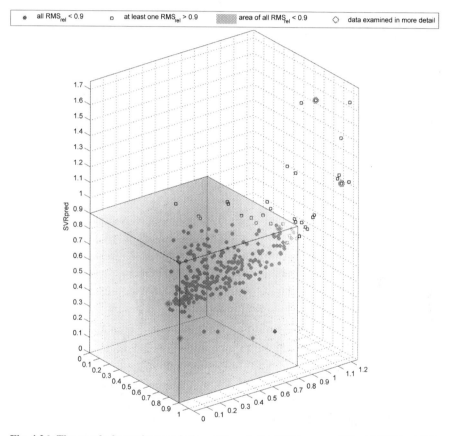

Fig. 4.26: The graph shows the correlation of the relative RMS errors of the MULIN, wLMS and SVRpred algorithms. One dot corresponds to the evaluation results of the three algorithms on one respiratory motion trace. Circles are those signals for which all algorithms delivered a prediction result with RMS$_{rel}$ below 0.9. The corresponding area is covered by the grey box. Each open square corresponds to a data set for wich at least one algorithm failed to deliver a result with RMS$_{rel} < 0.9$. Figure 4.27 shows the 2D projections of this graph.

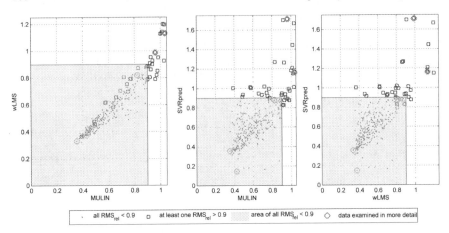

Fig. 4.27: Correlation of the relative RMS of the MULIN, wLMS and SVRpred algorithms, 2D projections of figure 4.26.

gnals are also corrupted by additional motion. The first 400 seconds of signals S1 to S4 are shown in figure 4.28.

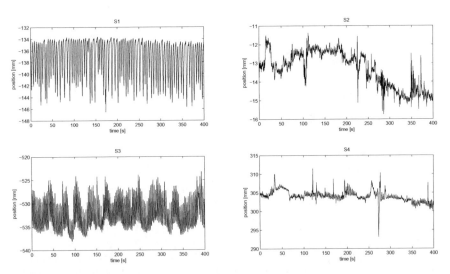

Fig. 4.28: Principal component of the motion trajectories of the signals S1 to S4, first 400 seconds. Note the regularity of S1 and S3 and the more random structure of S2 and S4.

4.5.3 Evaluation of the FLA-nLMS Algorithm

Since in section 4.5.2 the algorithm's optimal parameters were selected, the FLA-extension to the nLMS algorithm was omitted. This algorithm's main advantage is that it does not rely on optimal parameters due to its adaptation capabilities and it is thus evaluated in a somewhat different fashion:

For each signal, we used a grid search on the first 2,500 sampling points to find the locally optimal, and on the complete signal to find the globally optimal parameters μ and M. We then randomly selected 300 pairs of values of $(\mu, M) \in\,]0, 0.3] \times [1, 15]$ for each signal to test both the $nLMS_2$ and the $FLA\text{-}nLMS_2$ algorithms at $\sigma = 0.5$, $\tau = 0.95$, $A = 1500$, $L = 500$, $N = 31$. The resulting RMS error was then divided by the RMS error of the $nLMS_2$ predictor obtained using the locally optimal parameters for this signal. The results are shown in figure 4.29. Again, the fact that the

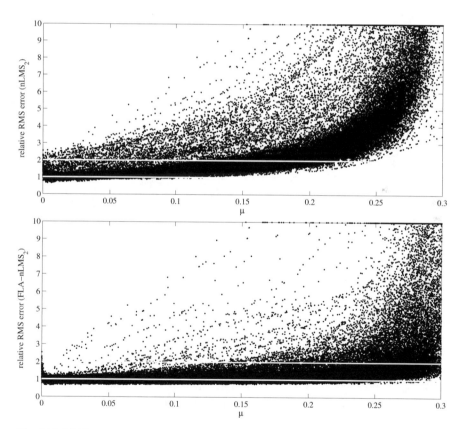

Fig. 4.29: RMS errors of evaluations of the $nLMS_2$ (top) and the $FLA\text{-}nLMS_2$ (bottom) algorithms using random values for μ and M, relative to the result obtained using locally optimal parameters. The light and dark grey lines indicate the 100 % and 200 % error levels, respectively.

nLMS$_2$ algorithm becomes unstable at some point can be observed clearly. On the other hand, the advantage of the FLA modification is obvious: the breakdown of the algorithm can be averted most of the time and the overall prediction performance increases. This is shown by the fact that the number of test cases with a relative RMS error of less than one is by far higher in the bottom part of figure 4.29.

A closer look at the raw data reveals that for more than 45 % of the 91,500 test cases, the relative RMS error comes to within ten percent of the value attainable using locally optimal parameters and for about 21 % even drops below it. When compared to the value obtained by using globally optimal parameters, these figures are reduced to 25 % and 2.5 %, respectively. In a second experiment, we tried seeding the FLA with the locally optimal values obtained after 96s (2,500 sampling points) of breathing. With this seeding, prediction errors on more than 98 % of the signals remained within ten percent of the value obtained using the locally optimal parameters and about 85 % even dropped below it. Again, using globally optimal parameters, these numbers decrease: to 92 % and 44 %, respectively. This can be seen in figure 4.30. Here, the following notational convention is used: 'gOpt' refers to the globally optimal and 'lOpt' to the locally optimal values for μ and M. 'seed' refers to the initial values used for μ_0 and M_0 in the algorithms. This shows that

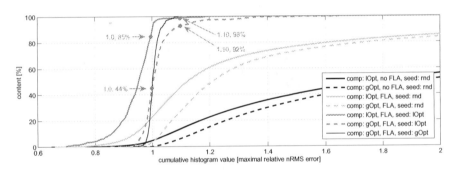

Fig. 4.30: Cumulative histogram of the relative RMS errors of the FLA-nLMS$_2$ algorithm on our database of 304 breathing motion signals

the FLA algorithm is capable of capturing changes in the breathing motion signal's dynamics and thus allows for a more stable prediction of the respiratory cycle. In fact, the prediction errors (relative to the mean signal amplitude) using this approach range from 2.99 % to 33.17 % with a mean of 8.30 %, whereas the mean prediction error obtained without the Fast Lane modification is 8.58 % (ranging from 3.11 % to 33.90 %). A complete overview is given in figure 4.31.

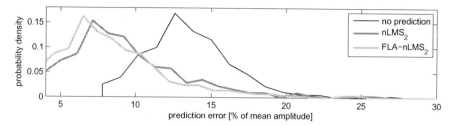

Fig. 4.31: Overview of the prediction errors of the nLMS$_2$ and the FLA-nLMS$_2$ relative to the mean signal amplitude

4.6 Predicting the Outcome of Prediction[6]

We now try to look for a method of quantifying the obvious differences between these signals. The first approach taken is based on the signals' Fourier transform. A 'good' respiratory motion trace is regular and should thus have a spectrum with prominent peaks and little DC drift. Figure 4.32 shows the spectra of the signals. We can clearly see that S1 and S3 do indeed have much more prominent peaks than S2 and S4. Furthermore, the energy levels of S1 and S3 are much higher than those of S2 and S4.

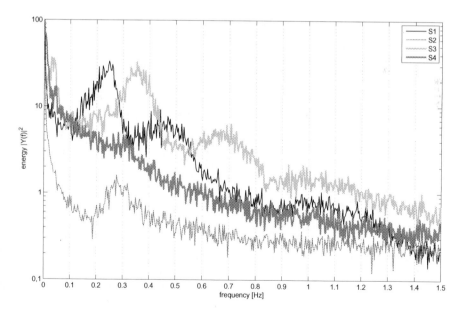

Fig. 4.32: Spectra of the signals S1 to S4

---

[6] Parts of this section have been published in [13].

To quantify these values, the signals' spectra were approximated by equation 4.27.

$$g(f) = \underbrace{a_0 \exp(a_1 f) + a_2}_{\text{exponential decay}} + \underbrace{\sum_{i=1}^{3} A_i \exp(-(f - \mu_i)^2/(2\sigma_i^2))}_{\text{three Gaussian peaks}} \qquad (4.27)$$

This function was selected to model the exponential decay, a possible low-frequency peak, the expected peak of the dominant respiratory frequency, and its first harmonic. The model was fitted to the power spectrum by minimising the RMS error between $|Y(f)|^2$ and $g(f)$, i.e., $\mathrm{RMS}\left(|Y(f)|^2 - g(f)\right) \to \min$. Optimal fitting was determined using MATLAB.

To actually compute the optimal fit, four functions were used:

$$\begin{aligned}
g_1(\mathbf{r}, f) &= r_1 \exp(r_2 f) + r_3 + r_4 \exp(-f^2/(2r_5^2)) \\
g_2(\mathbf{r}, f) &= g_1((r_1, \ldots, r_5)^{\mathrm{T}}, f) + r_6 \exp(-(f - r_7)^2/(2r_8^2)) \\
g_3(\mathbf{r}, f) &= g_2(x, f)\Big|_{x = \widehat{\mathbf{r}_2}} + r_1 \exp(-(f - r_2)^2/(2r_3^2)) \\
g_4(\mathbf{r}, f) &= g_2((r_1, \ldots, r_8)^{\mathrm{T}}, f) + r_9 \exp(-(f - r_{10})^2/(2r_{11}^2))
\end{aligned} \qquad (4.28)$$

where

$$\widehat{\mathbf{r}_i} = \operatorname*{argmin}_{\mathbf{r}} \mathrm{RMS}\left(|Y(f)|^2 - g_i(\mathbf{r}, f)\right).$$

Now the optimal parameters for equation 4.27 are computed as follows:

1. Determine $\widehat{\mathbf{r}_1}$ using the initial values $\mathbf{r} = (1, 0, 0, 1, 0.01)^{\mathrm{T}}$
2. Compute a smoothed version of the spectrum (this is done by taking a running average over 30 samples)
3. Determine the locations m_1 and m_2 of the first two peaks inside the range of 0.1 to 0.4 Hz of the smoothed spectrum. This is done using a thresholded min-max-search (see listing E.3 in appendix E) with $\tau = 0.15$.
4. Determine $\widehat{\mathbf{r}_2}$ using the initial values $\mathbf{r} = \left(\widehat{\mathbf{r}_1}^{\mathrm{T}}, 3, m_1, 0.005\right)^{\mathrm{T}}$. If no peaks were found in step two, m_1 is set to 0.25.
5. Determine $\widehat{\mathbf{r}_3}$ using the initial values $\mathbf{r} = (0.2(\widehat{\mathbf{r}_2})_6, m_2, (\widehat{\mathbf{r}_2})_8)^{\mathrm{T}}$. If no peaks or only one peak were found in step two, m_2 is set to $2(\widehat{\mathbf{r}_2})_7$.
6. Determine $\widehat{\mathbf{r}_4}$ by using the initial values $\mathbf{r} = \left(\widehat{\mathbf{r}_2}^{\mathrm{T}}, \widehat{\mathbf{r}_3}^{\mathrm{T}}\right)^{\mathrm{T}}$.

Optimisation is done in this fashion to ensure that Gaussian peaks are placed at the main frequency of respiration and its first harmonic, even if they are not very pronounced (this is the case for S2, see figure 4.32). Using this fitting approach, we now have a feature vector of twelve elements ($\widehat{\mathbf{r}_4}$ and $e = \mathrm{RMS}\left(|Y(f)|^2 - g_4(\widehat{\mathbf{r}_4}, f)\right)$) describing a signal's spectrum. Results of the fitting for the signals S1 to S4 are shown in figure 4.33.

As a second approach to determine a signal's characteristics, we looked at its autocorrelation for different delays. To this end, for a signal $y = (y_1, y_2, \ldots, y_N)^{\mathrm{T}}$, we

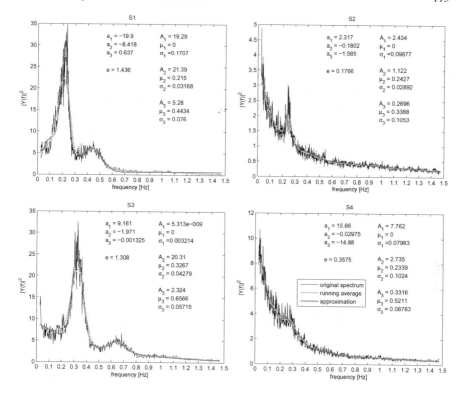

Fig. 4.33: Spectra of the four signals S1 to S4 (black), running average over 30 samples (light grey), and fitted function (dark grey). Additionally, the fitting parameters a_1 to a_3 and A_i, μ_i, σ_i, $i = 1, \ldots, 3$ and the fitting error e are shown.

computed the signal $r = (r_1, r_2, \ldots, r_{200})^{\mathrm{T}}$, the first 200 values of y's autocorrelation function. Assume that

$$\bar{y}_{i,j} = \frac{1}{N - i - j} \sum_{n=1+i}^{N-j} y_n.$$

Then the components of r are computed as

$$r_k = \frac{\sum_{i=1}^{N-k} (y_{i+k} - \bar{y}_{k,0})(y_i - \bar{y}_{0,k})}{\sqrt{\sum_{i=1}^{5000-k} (y_{i+k} - \bar{y}_{k,0})^2 \sum_{i=1}^{N-k} (y_i - \bar{y}_{0,k})^2}}, \quad k = 1, \ldots, 200. \qquad (4.29)$$

Here, N is an arbitrary, but suitably large, number. We used $N = 5000$ in our experiments. We expect that signals well-suited to prediction should show strong periodicity in the autocorrelation function. To capture this behaviour in numbers, two functions to model r are computed. The first function is a simple linear fit, i.e.,

$$r_k^{\text{linear}} = m \cdot k \cdot T_s + t, \quad k = 1, \dots, 200, \tag{4.30}$$

where m and t are selected such that $\text{RMS}\left(r - r^{\text{linear}}\right) \to \min$. Here, T_s is the temporal spacing of the signal's samples. The residual error $\text{RMS}\left(r - r^{\text{linear}}\right)$ will be called e_{lin}.

The second function tries to model the autocorrelation function as a tapered cosine on top of the linear fit, i.e.,

$$r_k^{\cos} = r_k^{\text{linear}} + A \cdot \cos\left(\frac{2\pi}{T} \cdot k \cdot T_s\right)\left(1 + a_1 \cdot k \cdot T_s + a_2\left(k \cdot T_s\right)^2\right). \tag{4.31}$$

Here, the parameters A (amplitude), T (period length), a_1 and a_2 (tapering coefficients) are selected such that $\text{RMS}\left(r - r^{\cos}\right) \to \min$. The residual RMS error $\text{RMS}\left(r - r^{\cos}\right)$ will be called $e_{\cos}$.

The autocorrelation functions r, the resulting fits r^{linear} and $r^{\cos}$, and the corresponding parameters for the signals S1 to S4 are shown in figure 4.34.

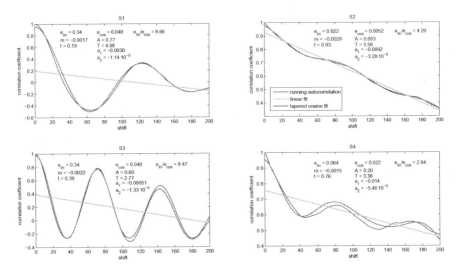

Fig. 4.34: Autocorrelation function of the signals S1 to S4 and the fitted functions r^{linear} and $r^{\cos}$, their residual errors, and the corresponding parameters m, t, A, T, a_1, and a_2.

Using both the autocorrelation and frequency fitting approaches, we can now determine a total of 21 features for each signal: nine from the autocorrelation fit and twelve from the frequency fit. To determine the features of an arbitrary signal, a MATLAB GUI was developed (see figure 4.35).

This analysis was done on all 304 signals to generate the corresponding feature vectors. The main goal now is to determine the correlation between the features and the prediction error on the signal. Table 4.8 shows the correlation coefficients between the individual features and the relative RMS errors of the prediction algorithms.

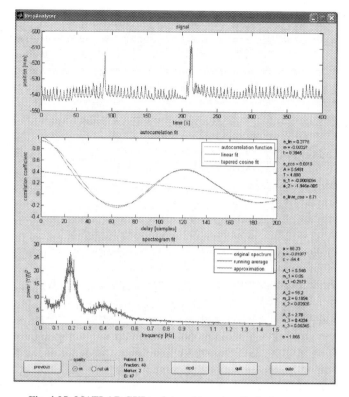

Fig. 4.35: MATLAB GUI to determine a signal's feature vector

Table 4.8: Correlation coefficients between the signal features and the relative RMS error of the prediction algorithms. Items marked in bold have correlation coefficients $|\rho| \geq 0.3$.

(a) Autocorrelation

algorithm	e_{lin}	m	t	e_{cos}	A	T	a_1	a_2	e_{lin}/e_{cos}
MULIN	**-0.30**	0.00	**0.37**	-0.05	-0.26	-0.00	0.01	-0.03	-0.21
nLMS	-0.28	-0.01	**0.33**	-0.13	-0.17	-0.11	0.07	-0.08	-0.20
RLS	-0.26	0.01	0.28	-0.05	-0.19	-0.04	0.03	-0.04	-0.23
wLMS	**-0.37**	-0.01	**0.48**	-0.06	**-0.34**	0.03	0.02	-0.02	-0.24
EKF	**-0.33**	-0.05	**0.43**	0.02	-0.30	0.15	0.00	0.01	-0.30
SVRpred	**-0.36**	-0.02	**0.50**	-0.09	**-0.33**	0.05	0.04	-0.04	-0.17

(b) Spectrogram

algorithm	a_1	a_2	a_3	A_1	σ_1	A_2	μ_2	σ_2	A_3	μ_1	σ_3	e
MULIN	0.04	-0.04	-0.05	0.01	0.01	**-0.65**	-0.05	-0.07	**-0.31**	0.11	0.00	**-0.53**
nLMS	0.06	-0.08	-0.06	0.01	0.00	**-0.41**	0.15	0.06	-0.02	0.19	0.00	-0.29
RLS	0.03	-0.06	-0.03	-0.01	-0.01	**-0.59**	0.01	-0.04	-0.21	0.11	0.03	**-0.48**
wLMS	0.03	-0.03	-0.03	0.02	0.01	**-0.65**	-0.07	-0.06	-0.30	0.07	0.01	**-0.51**
EKF	0.09	-0.04	-0.06	-0.03	-0.05	**-0.49**	-0.24	0.11	-0.09	-0.11	0.04	-0.22
SVRpred	0.08	0.02	-0.08	0.00	-0.01	**-0.49**	-0.10	-0.02	-0.25	0.04	0.01	**-0.35**

Looking at this data shows that six out of the 21 features show a correlation coefficient of at least 0.3 to the relative RMS error of one algorithm in at least one case: e_{lin}, t, A, A_2, A_3, and e. To determine how independent these features are, the correlation coefficients between them were also computed. The results are given in table 4.9.

Table 4.9: Correlation coefficients of the six dominant features

	e_{lin}	t	A	A_2	A_3	e
e_{lin}	1.000	-0.771	0.819	0.253	0.207	0.178
t	-0.771	1.000	-0.775	-0.332	-0.238	-0.234
A	0.819	-0.775	1.000	0.302	0.220	0.166
A_2	0.253	-0.332	0.302	1.000	0.577	0.752
A_3	0.207	-0.238	0.220	0.577	1.000	0.466
e	0.178	-0.234	0.166	0.752	0.466	1.000

This shows that, while the features from the autocorrelation fit and the spectrum fit show high correlation, their mutual correlation is much lower: below 0.3 in all but two cases.

We now turn to classifying the respiratory signals' prediction errors using the six dominant features identified. To simulate realistic settings, the features were recomputed on the first 7,800 samples (i.e., approximately 300 seconds) of the signals. Then, for each pair of dominant features, a 2D colour/shape-coded plot was created (shown in figure 4.36). The dots in these plots show the relation of the respective features and the dots' colours/shapes show the relative RMS errors of the MULIN algorithm: red squares correspond to a relative RMS of one or more, green diamonds correspond to $0.9 \leq \text{RMS}_{\text{rel}} < 1$, blue crosses correspond to $0.8 \leq \text{RMS}_{\text{rel}} < 0.9$, and black circles are signals with $\text{RMS}_{\text{rel}} < 0.8$. Then, for each plot, a polygon (shown in magenta) was drawn. This polygon should, by decreasing priority,

1. contain as many red squares as possible and
2. as many green diamonds as possible and
3. as many blue crosses as possible and
4. as few black circles as possible,
5. while having the smallest possible area and being as close to rectangular as possible.

Then the number of points inside (circles) or outside (squares, diamonds, crosses) the polygon was computed. These numbers are shown as "incorrectly classified" in each plot. It is now also possible to extend the constraints for classification: instead of using one polygon only (as was done in plots (a) to (o) of figure 4.36), we reject a signal (i.e., assume that its relative RMS will be ≥ 0.8) if it is contained in at least n polygons:

> A signal s will be rejected if there are at least n feature pairs which are contained in the corresponding polygons.

Using this approach for all $n \in \{1, 2, \ldots, 15\}$, plot (p) of figure 4.36 was generated. This plot shows that, for increasing n (i.e., the required feature pairs), the number of incorrectly rejected signals (black circles) decreases while the share of falsely accepted signals (blue crosses, green diamonds, and red squares) increases.

Typically, signals resulting in a relative RMS of more than 1 (red curve with squares) must be rejected, signals with relative RMS between 0.9 and 1 should be rejected, and signals with relative RMS between 0.8 and 0.9 can be rejected. Unfortunately, the classification errors are still quite high: when using $n = 6$, 11 % of all acceptable signals will be incorrectly rejected, 52 % of the "can"-signals and 36 % of the "should"-signals will be falsely accepted.

To further reduce these numbers, a second classifier is introduced. Since the MULIN algorithms are very fast, it is possible to optimise the algorithms' parameters on the short signal sequence used to compute classification.

The correspondence between the relative RMS of the short signal and the relative RMS of the full signal is shown in figure 4.37a. Here, black dots are correctly classified points (based on the 0.8 cutoff line), whereas red crosses mark incorrectly classified signals.

We can see that basing classification exclusively on the values of the optimal relative RMS on the short signals is also error-prone. While incorrect rejection is rare (only three signals, i.e., 1.2 %), false acceptance is comparable to the levels of the original classification approach. This leads to the idea of incorporating the MULIN classification data into the original algorithm:

> A signal s will be rejected if there are at least n feature pairs which are contained in the corresponding polygons **or** the evaluation of the MULIN algorithm on the first five minutes shows a relative RMS of more than 0.8.

While this combination will not reduce the number of incorrect rejections, it will change the probability of falsely accepting a signal. The resulting graphs are given in figure 4.37b. We can see that the false acceptance rates have dropped considerably whereas the false rejection rate has not changed much. For six and nine feature pairs as well as for the MULIN classifier alone, the numbers are given in table 4.10.

This shows us that it is feasible to predict—with acceptable accuracy—whether a patient's respiratory motion trace will be suitable for prediction or not.

This classification has now also been applied to both the wLMS and SVRpred algorithms. To reduce the possibility of overfitting the classifier, the same polygons as used for the MULIN classification were used. The results are convincing: the classification errors for both algorithms, computed without using the prediction quality on the short sub-signal, are close to those obtained for the MULIN algorithms. Including the prediction error on the sub-signal will, in both cases, significantly decrease the false acceptance rates, in the case of the wLMS algorithm, all signals

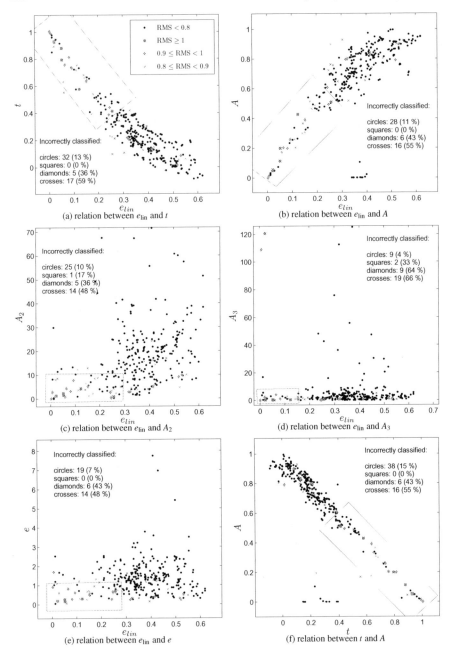

(a) relation between e_{lin} and t

(b) relation between e_{lin} and A

(c) relation between e_{lin} and A_2

(d) relation between e_{lin} and A_3

(e) relation between e_{lin} and e

(f) relation between t and A

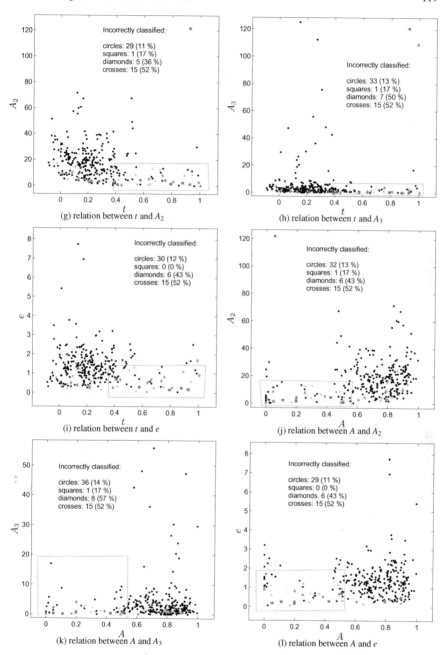

(g) relation between t and A_2

(h) relation between t and A_3

(i) relation between t and e

(j) relation between A and A_2

(k) relation between A and A_3

(l) relation between A and e

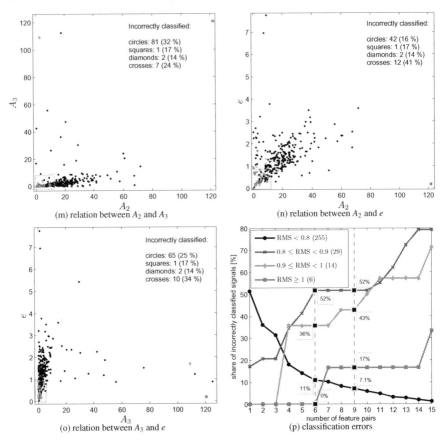

Fig. 4.36: Classification of signals according to their features

Table 4.10: Classification errors for the MULIN algorithm

classifier	RMS < 0.8	0.8 ≤ RMS < 0.9	0.9 ≤ RMS < 1	RMS ≥ 1
polygon, without prediction results on short signal				
6FP	11.0 %	51.7 %	35.7 %	—
9FP	7.1 %	51.7 %	42.9 %	16.7 %
based only on prediction results on short signal				
	1.2 %	37.9 %	35.7 %	—
polygon, including prediction results on short signal				
6FP	11.4 %	13.8 %	14.3 %	—
9FP	7.5 %	13.8 %	21.4 %	—
number of signals				
	255	29	14	6

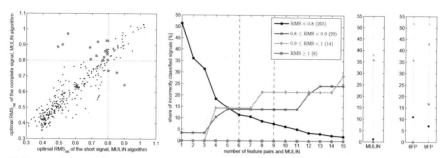

(a) Correspondence between the optimal relative RMS computed on the short signal and the optimal RMS on the complete signal.

(b) Errors of the modified classification method (left), classification errors of the data from figure 4.37a (centre), and classification errors of the original classification method for six and nine feature pairs from figure 4.36 (right).

Fig. 4.37: Classification of signals according to their features, including prediction error on a short part of the signal

with $RMS_{rel} \geq 0.9$ are rejected. Very noticeable, however, is the fact that the SVR-pred's false rejectance rate increases dramatically when the additional prediction error is used as classifier. Looking at figure 4.27 gives a possible explanation: since classification works very well for both the MULIN and wLMS methods, and the RMS errors of these methods are not very much correlated to the RMS errors of the SVRpred algorithm, it is reasonable to assume that, for the SVRpred method, other features might be more important. Looking at table 4.8 shows us that, for both the MULIN and wLMS methods, the correlation between the dominant features and the RMS error is more than 0.5 in two of the six cases. For the SVRpred algorithm, however, it is always below 0.5.

The complete classification results are given in table 4.11 (wLMS) and table 4.12 (SVRpred).

Table 4.11: Classification errors for the wLMS algorithm

classifier	RMS < 0.8	$0.8 \leq RMS < 0.9$	$0.9 \leq RMS < 1$	RMS ≥ 1
polygon, without prediction results on short signal				
6FP	10.7 %	20.0 %	—	—
9FP	7.0 %	25.0 %	—	16.7 %
based only on prediction results on short signal				
	2.4 %	75.9 %	50.0 %	—
polygon, including prediction results on short signal				
6FP	12.9 %	15.0 %	—	—
9FP	9.2 %	20.0 %	—	—
number of signals				
	272	20	6	6

Table 4.12: Classification errors for the SVRpred algorithm

classifier	RMS < 0.8	0.8 ≤ RMS < 0.9	0.9 ≤ RMS < 1	RMS ≥ 1
polygon, without prediction results on short signal				
6FP	9.3 %	53.3 %	33.3 %	20.0 %
9FP	5.7 %	53.3 %	41.7 %	33.3 %
based only on prediction results on short signal				
	25.1 %	41.4 %	14.3 %	—
polygon, including prediction results on short signal				
6FP	26.3 %	26.7 %	25.0 %	—
9FP	23.9 %	26.7 %	25.0 %	—
number of signals				
	247	30	12	15

4.7 Prediction of Human Pulsatory Motion[7]

While the algorithms presented in this chapter have been developed with applicability to respiratory motion prediction in mind, it is conceivable to also apply them to human pulsatory motion traces. The CyberHeart project (see section 2.5) has sparked interest in live compensation of cardiac motion with a robotic device. Consequently, we have evaluated the applicability of the aforementioned algorithms to cardiac 3D motion traces.

They are evaluated on actual cardiac motion traces recorded with 3D Ultrasound (US), the NavX(M) catheter system and optical tracking of the cardiac apex beat. How this data was acquired is explained in more detail in section 4.7.1. In section 4.7.2 we show that this prediction is actually possible and that the results are very convincing.

4.7.1 Data Acquisition

To test the prediction algorithms, we used test data from several modalities. These were:

1. Externally measured motion of the apex cordis
2. Internally measured motion using the EnSite NavX catheter system
3. Internally measured motion using 3D US

All externally measured data and all US data was acquired in our laboratory from healthy probands. The NavX data was provided by courtesy of CyberHeart, Inc.

It is clear that the motion traces recorded externally as well as the motion traces recorded using US do not necessarily represent the motion of the target area. In this work, however, we are looking at the feasibility of applying prediction algorithms

---

[7] Parts of this section have been published in [8, 19]

to cardiac motion. As a consequence, it is insightful to look at motion recorded at different anatomical sites using different imaging or tracking modalities.

From [35] we know that the prediction algorithms currently used clinically in the CyberKnife all work on one-dimensional data. To successfully compensate for three-dimensional motion, however, three separate prediction algorithms have to be used, one for each spatial dimension of the internal target motion. To simplify the evaluation process, it is commonplace to only consider the surrogate's principal component of motion. We have also resorted to this approach for the ultrasonic and externally acquired data. Since the NavX motion traces have been recorded with high precision inside the beating heart, we have, in this case, analysed all three spatial directions.

In clinical reality, the methodology would be to track the cardiac motion signal in three dimensions and to analyse the first couple of seconds of the signal to find it's principal component and the matrix describing this transformation. Then three prediction algorithms are run on the signal after applying the transformation matrix.

Externally measured motion

In a first experiment, we attached a custom-built LED net (presented in [25]) to the chest of nine healthy male volunteers (ages 22 to 31 years) and recorded a total of 16 datasets. We made sure that multiple LEDs covered the left fifth intercostal space to be able to record the heart's apex beat. The LEDs were tracked using the accuTrack 250 system which has a very high temporal (4.1 kHz single LED sampling rate) and spatial resolution. The camera was placed approximately 30 cm away from the LED net. The probands were asked to hold their breath to record a motion trace of the apex cordis (shown in figure 4.38). The sampling rates of the experiments ranged from 100 to 780 Hz, depending on the number of LEDs actually tracked.

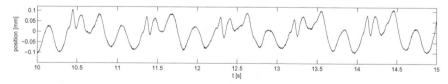

Fig. 4.38: Principal component of the motion of the apex cordis as recorded by an LED placed in the left fifth intercostal space, tracked under breath hold by the accuTrack 250 system.

All external signals were processed to remove baseline drift from proband motion other than respiration or pulsation. This was done by subtracting a running average from the actual signal. Note that in clinical reality, this approach is not feasible, but since the purpose of this work is to demonstrate the applicability of respiratory motion prediction algorithms to pulsatory motion, we have, in this case, decided to forego direct clinical reproducibility.

Internally measured motion

We used two different types of internally measured signals. The first was acquired using an EnSite NavX catheter system. Using this device, it is possible to compute the position of the NavX catheter inside the heart based on measurements of an electrical field created on the patient's chest. The data was acquired during normal heart rhythm of a 60-year-old male undergoing ablation treatment for paroxysmal atrial fibrillation. The patient was in narcosis and five datasets were collected. The reference catheter was placed in the sinus cavity and an SPL catheter was placed in the left inferior pulmonary vein (one data set), the right superior pulmonary vein (two data sets) and the left superior pulmonary vein (two datasets). The SPL catheter consists of 20 electrodes the position data of which was averaged to determine the motion of the pulmonary vein's centroid. The five datasets are all about 30 s long. The principal component of motion of one electrode is shown in figure 4.39.

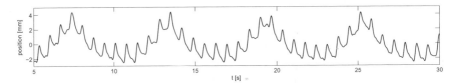

Fig. 4.39: Principal component of motion of one electrode as recorded by the NavX system (92 Hz).

The second signal was recorded in our laboratory using a GE Vivid7 Dimension[(N)] US station, using a 3V 3D/4D transducer for cardiac imaging. The transducer was attached to an industrial robot, adept Viper s850, and subsequently placed such as to generate a four chamber view of the heart (see figure 4.41). Using the method presented in [3], we tracked the position of the septum for approximately six minutes. Although the data recorded is a 3D trajectory, due to the poor resolution of the transducer, we could not perform prediction in all three spatial axes of the signal. We therefore reduced the signal to its principal component of motion, which is shown in figure 4.40.
We recorded a total of ten signals from six volunteers (five male, one female), all without cardiac arrhythmia.

4.7.2 Results

We have evaluated the test signals using the following prediction algorithms: EKF, nLMS, wLMS, MULIN, and SVRpred. The prediction horizon was set to 120 ms, which is approximately the prediction horizon required for the CyberKnife system. Evaluation was done using the relative RMS of the predicted signal as a measure of quality, see definition 2.

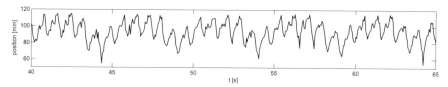

Fig. 4.40: Principal component of the septum's motion as recorded in 3D US using template matching (18 Hz).

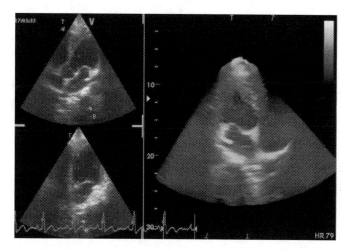

Fig. 4.41: Ultrasonic view of the heart as used to measure the motion of the septum

The algorithms' parameters were selected such as to generate a prediction with minimal relative RMS. The evaluation was done using the prediction toolkit (see section 4.4) and a simple grid search algorithm.

The results are shown in figure 4.42 and table 4.13. We have been able to successfully predict all signals, some better, and some worse. Most noticeable, however, is the fact that there is no prediction algorithm which is optimal for all signals. While the SVRpred algorithm performs best on 28 of the 41 signals (68.3 % of the signals), it is beaten by the EKF approach in seven cases (17.1 %), by the nLMS algorithm in three cases (7.3 %), by the wLMS algorithm in two cases (4.9 %) and by the MU-LIN algorithms in one case (2.4 %). While the difference between the relative RMS of the SVRpred algorithm and the one outperforming it is usually small (mean of 0.0721, median of 0.0456), it can be much higher: more than 0.1 in three cases and more than 0.3 once. Note that in this extreme case, SVRpred failed to deliver a functioning prediction: its optimal relative RMS was 1.091. The complete data is shown in figure 4.43a.

In general, it seems that it doesn't matter much which source and anatomical region the signal comes from: in most cases, it was possible to get a prediction with relative RMS below 0.75, in many cases even below 0.5. A slight advantage seems to lie with the externally measured data, possibly due to their high spatial and temporal

Table 4.13: Performance of the individual algorithms. Read: on the NavX datasets, the SVR-pred algorithm performed best on 11 out of the 15 datasets.

	MULIN	nLMS	EKF	wLMS	SVRpred
external data (16)	—	3	1	—	12
US data (10)	1	—	4	—	5
NavX data (15)	—	—	2	2	11
all (41)	1	3	7	2	28

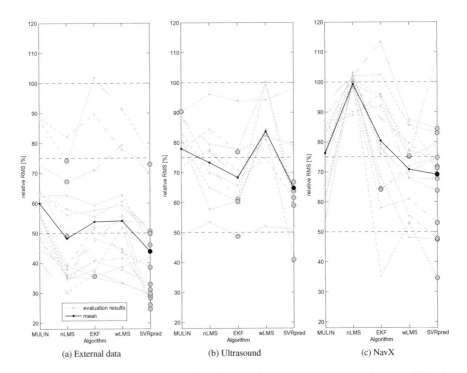

(a) External data   (b) Ultrasound   (c) NavX

Fig. 4.42: Results of the prediction algorithms. Each grey curve corresponds to one dataset. The large dots mark the algorithm with the best performance. The black curve represents the average performance of the algorithms.

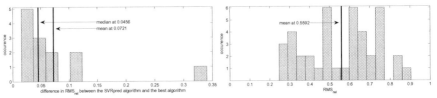

(a) Histogram of the differences in relative RMS between the SVRpred algorithm and the algorithm outperforming the SVRpred algorithm

(b) Relative RMS of the optimal prediction algorithm

Fig. 4.43: Histograms showing the performance of the SVRpred algorithm

resolution. The relative RMS error ranges from 0.247 to 0.904 with a mean of 0.559. More details are shown in figure 4.43b.

The results clearly show that it is advantageous to predict the motion signals to decrease the robot's latency since the error can be reduced by as much as 75 %. Furthermore, it would be interesting to analyse whether it is possible to increase the accuracy of prediction by first breaking down the signal into respiratory and pulsatory motion. These signals could then be predicted on their own and merged afterwards. It is clear that, although it is the most complex and flexible algorithm, the SVRpred method is not always optimal: it might not work at all and may be outperformed by other, simpler algorithms. It is interesting, however, that both the EKF and the nLMS algorithm have been shown to be inferior in performance to the SVRpred, the MULIN and the wLMS algorithm when it comes to prediction of respiratory signals (see section 4.5). The likely reason is that cardiac motion is completely involuntary and hence more regular.

It must be noted, however, that in reality we will not deal with patients with normal heartbeat: the system is intended to be used to cure atrial fibrillation and we thus cannot expect their pulsatory motion to be as regular as the motion of healthy probands. The approach which could be followed clinically would be to medically suppress atrial fibrillation for the duration of the treatment and to continuously monitor the patient's cardiac activity using Electrocardiogram (ECG). Should the ECG show that the patient is about to develop cardiac arrhythmia, or should the motion compensation system detect anomalous motion patterns, the treatment beam would have to be switched off until the patient's cardiac motion comes back to normal.

Further possible applications of cardiac motion prediction are all operations on the beating heart, being an alternative to operations under cardiopulmonary bypass. Moreover, the so called On-Pump-technique often results in cognitive disruptions. Accurate prediction of cardiac motion could be able to synchronise surgical devices to the heart to avoid suppression of the natural heartbeat. One possible application has been described in [42].

References

[1] ALGLIB – a cross-platform numerical analysis and data processing library. Available online. URL http://www.alglib.net

[2] Bartz, D., Bohn, S., Hoffmann, J. (eds.): Jahrestagung der Deutschen Gesellschaft für Computer- und Roboterassistierte Chirurgie, vol. 7. CURAC, Leipzig, Germany (2008)

[3] Bruder, R., Ernst, F., Schlaefer, A., Schweikard, A.: Real-time tracking of the pulmonary veins in 3D ultrasound of the beating heart. In: 51st Annual Meeting of the AAPM, *Medical Physics*, vol. 36, p. 2804. American Association of Physicists in Medicine, Anaheim, CA, USA (2009). DOI 10.1118/1.3182643. TH-C-304A-07

[4] CMake cross-platform build tools. Available online. URL http://www.cmake.org

[5] Demartines, P., Herault, J.: Curvilinear component analysis: a self-organizing neural networkfor nonlinear mapping of data sets. IEEE Transactions on Neural Networks **8**(1), 148–154 (1997). DOI 10.1109/72.554199

[6] Dieterich, S.: Private communication (Mar., 2008, and Oct., 2010)

[7] Douglas, S.C.: A family of normalized LMS algorithms. IEEE Signal Processing Letters **1**(3), 49–55 (1994)

[8] Ernst, F., Bruder, R., Pohl, M., Schlaefer, A., Schweikard, A.: Prediction of cardiac motion. In: Proceedings of the 24th International Conference and Exhibition on Computer Assisted Radiology and Surgery (CARS'10), *International Journal of CARS*, vol. 5, pp. 273–274. CARS, Geneva, Switzerland (2010)

[9] Ernst, F., Bruder, R., Schlaefer, A.: Processing of respiratory signals from tracking systems for motion compensated IGRT. In: 49th Annual Meeting of the AAPM, *Medical Physics*, vol. 34, p. 2565. American Association of Physicists in Medicine, Minneapolis-St. Paul, MN, USA (2007). DOI 10.1118/1.2761413. TU-EE-A3-4

[10] Ernst, F., Schlaefer, A., Dieterich, S., Schweikard, A.: A fast lane approach to LMS prediction of respiratory motion signals. Biomedical Signal Processing and Control **3**(4), 291–299 (2008). DOI 10.1016/j.bspc.2008.06.001

[11] Ernst, F., Schlaefer, A., Schweikard, A.: Prediction of respiratory motion with wavelet-based multiscale autoregression. In: N. Ayache, S. Ourselin, A. Maeder (eds.) MICCAI 2007, Part II, *Lecture Notes in Computer Science*, vol. 4792, pp. 668–675. MICCAI, Springer, Brisbane, Australia (2007). DOI 10.1007/978-3-540-75759-7_81

[12] Ernst, F., Schlaefer, A., Schweikard, A.: Processing of respiratory motion traces for motion-compensated radiotherapy. Medical Physics **37**(1), 282–294 (2010). DOI 10.1118/1.3271684

[13] Ernst, F., Schlaefer, A., Schweikard, A.: Predicting the outcome of respiratory motion prediction. Medical Physics **38**(10), accepted for publication (2011)

[14] Ernst, F., Schweikard, A.: A family of linear algorithms for the prediction of respiratory motion in image-guided radiotherapy. In: Proceedings of the 22nd International Conference and Exhibition on Computer Assisted Radiology and Surgery (CARS'08), *International Journal of CARS*, vol. 3, pp. 31–32. CARS, Barcelona, Spain (2008). DOI 10.1007/s11548-008-0169-x

[15] Ernst, F., Schweikard, A.: Predicting respiratory motion signals for image-guided radiotherapy using multi-step linear methods (MULIN). International Journal of Computer Assisted Radiology and Surgery **3**(1–2), 85–90 (2008). DOI 10.1007/s11548-008-0211-z

[16] Ernst, F., Schweikard, A.: Prediction of respiratory motion using a modified Recursive Least Squares algorithm. In: Bartz et al. [2], pp. 157–160

[17] Ernst, F., Schweikard, A.: Forecasting respiratory motion with accurate online support vector regression (SVRpred). International Journal of Computer

Assisted Radiology and Surgery **4**(5), 439–447 (2009). DOI 10.1007/s11548-009-0355-5

[18] Ernst, F., Schweikard, A.: Predicting respiratory motion signals using accurate online support vector regression (SVRpred). In: Proceedings of the 23rd International Conference and Exhibition on Computer Assisted Radiology and Surgery (CARS'09), *International Journal of CARS*, vol. 4, pp. 255–256. CARS, Berlin, Germany (2009). DOI 10.1007/s11548-009-0340-z

[19] Ernst, F., Stender, B., Schlaefer, A., Schweikard, A.: Using ECG in motion prediction for radiosurgery of the beating heart. In: G.Z. Yang, A. Darzi (eds.) The Hamlyn Symposium on Medical Robotics, vol. 3, pp. 37–38 (2010)

[20] Griffiths, L.J.: A simple adaptive algorithm for real-time processing in antenna arrays. Proceedings of the IEEE **57**(10), 1696–1704 (1969)

[21] Hager, W.W., Zhang, H.: A new active set algorithm for box constrained optimization. SIAM Journal on Optimization **17**(2), 526–557 (2006). DOI 10.1137/050635225

[22] Haykin, S.: Adaptive Filter Theory, 4th edn. Prentice Hall, Englewood Cliffs, NJ (2002)

[23] Kalman, R.E.: A new approach to linear filtering and prediction problems. Transactions of the ASME Journal of Basic Engineering **82D**, 35–45 (1960)

[24] Kalman, R.E., Bucy, R.S.: New results in linear filtering and prediction theory. Transactions of the ASME Journal of Basic Engineering **83D**, 95–108 (1961)

[25] Knöpke, M., Ernst, F.: Flexible Markergeometrien zur Erfassung von Atmungs- und Herzbewegungen an der Körperoberfläche. In: Bartz et al. [2], pp. 15–16

[26] Lee, J.A., Lendasse, A., Verleysen, M.: Curvilinear distance analysis versus isomap. In: European Symposium on Artificial Neural Networks (ESANN), pp. 185–192. Bruges (Belgium) (2002)

[27] Ma, J., Theiler, J., Perkins, S.: Accurate on-line support vector regression. Neural Computation **15**(11), 2683–2703 (2003). DOI 10.1162/089976603322385117

[28] McCall, K.C., Jeraj, R.: Dual-component model of respiratory motion based on the periodic autoregressive moving average (periodic ARMA) method. Physics in Medicine and Biology **52**(12), 3455–3466 (2007). DOI 10.1088/0031-9155/52/12/009

[29] Parrella, F.: Online support vector regression. Master's thesis, University of Genoa (2007)

[30] Ramrath, L., Schlaefer, A., Ernst, F., Dieterich, S., Schweikard, A.: Prediction of respiratory motion with a multi-frequency based Extended Kalman Filter. In: Proceedings of the 21st International Conference and Exhibition on Computer Assisted Radiology and Surgery (CARS'07), *International Journal of CARS*, vol. 2, pp. 56–58. CARS, Berlin, Germany (2007). DOI 10.1007/s11548-007-0083-7

[31] Ren, Q., Nishioka, S., Shirato, H., Berbeco, R.I.: Adaptive prediction of respiratory motion for motion compensation radiotherapy. Physics in Medicine and Biology **52**(22), 6651–6661 (2007). DOI 10.1088/0031-9155/52/22/007

[32] Renaud, O., Starck, J.L., Murtagh, F.: Prediction based on a multiscale decomposition. International Journal of Wavelets, Multiresolution and Information Processing 1(2), 217–232 (2003)

[33] Renaud, O., Starck, J.L., Murtagh, F.: Wavelet-based combined signal filtering and prediction. IEEE Transactions on Systems, Man and Cybernetics, Part B: Cybernetics 35(6), 1241–1251 (2005)

[34] Rzezovski, N., Ernst, F.: Graphical tool for the prediction of respiratory motion signals. In: Bartz et al. [2], pp. 179–180

[35] Sayeh, S., Wang, J., Main, W.T., Kilby, W., Maurer Jr., C.R.: Robotic Radiosurgery. Treating Tumors that Move with Respiration, 1st edn., chap. Respiratory motion tracking for robotic radiosurgery, pp. 15–30. Springer, Berlin (2007). DOI 10.1007/978-3-540-69886-9

[36] Sheng, Y., Li, S., Sayeh, S., Wang, J., Wang, H.: Fuzzy and hybrid prediction of position signal in SynchronyÂ® respiratory tracking system. In: R.J.P. de Figueiredo (ed.) SIP 2007, pp. 459–464. IASTED, Acta Press, Honolulu, USA (2007)

[37] Tenenbaum, J.B., de Silva, V., Langford, J.C.: A global geometric framework for nonlinear dimensionality reduction. Science 290, 2319–2323 (2000)

[38] Vedam, S.S., Keall, P.J., Docef, A., Todor, D.A., Kini, V.R., Mohan, R.: Predicting respiratory motion for four-dimensional radiotherapy. Medical Physics 31(8), 2274–2283 (2004). DOI 10.1118/1.1771931

[39] Verleysen, M., Francois, D.: The curse of dimensionality in data mining and time series prediction. In: Proceedings of the 8th International Workshop on Artificial Neural Networks (IWANN 2005), Lecture Notes in Computer Science, vol. 3512, pp. 758–770. Springer, Barcelona, Spain (2005). DOI 10.1007/11494669_93

[40] Widrow, B., Hoff, M.E.: Adaptive switching circuits. In: IRE WESCON Convention Record, vol. 4, pp. 96–104 (1960)

[41] wxWidgets – a cross-platform GUI library. Available online. URL http://www.wxwidgets.org

[42] Yuen, S.G., Kettler, D.T., Novotny, P.M., Plowes, R.D., Howe, R.D.: Robotic motion compensation for beating heart intracardiac surgery. International Journal of Robotics Research 28(10), 1355–1372 (2009). DOI 10.1177/0278364909104065

Chapter 5
Going Inside: Correlation between External and Internal Respiratory Motion[1]

In an ideal setting, the target area could be located directly using a non-invasive, high resolution, high speed tracking or imaging modality. Currently, however, there is no single device capable of meeting all these demands. Options available are either invasive, like biplanar fluoroscopy [34–38] or EM tracking [2, 20, 41], are still under development, like US tracking [13, 29, 42], live Magnetic Resonance Imaging (MRI) [17, 21, 26, 27] or monoscopic fluoroscopy [3, 4], or require correlation between external signals and sparsely recorded internal data [23, 25, 32, 33].

Since most of these technologies are not yet available clinically (like live MRI, US tracking, or monoscopic fluoroscopy), cannot be used universally (like EM-tracking) or are too invasive (like real-time biplanar fluoroscopy), the main focus is placed on hybrid methods which require external surrogates to fill the gaps between less frequently acquired internal data.

5.1 Correlation Algorithms

The correlation between surrogate motion and target motion has been evaluated in [1, 11, 19], linear correlation algorithms have been proposed and evaluated in [12, 14, 15, 24, 30–32, 39], more complex models based on Neural Networks [14, 24, 43], Support Vector Regression [9], Kalman Filtering [14, 24] and PCA [16] have also been evaluated. Another approach is to classify respiratory motion and fit a general model. This has been done in [10], where sinusoidal models were evaluated. A more generic respiratory model using 4D-CT data has been created in [22]. Recently, a new look has been taken at monoscopic X-ray instead of the commonly used bi-planar fluoroscopic approach [3, 4]. In this work, we focus on simple polynomial correlation as outlined in [30] and on Support Vector Regression as proposed in [9].

---

[1] Parts of this chapter have been published in [8, 9]

General Assumptions

To outline possible correlation algorithms, we assume the following situation: radio-opaque markers (i.e., gold fiducials) are visualised using a biplanar fluoroscopy system. At the same time, the positions of externally visible markers (i.e., Infrared (IR) LEDs) are recorded using a tracking system. For the sake of clarity, we assume the recording of the fiducial and LED positions to occur simultaneously.

Let us assume that N is the number of samples we have taken. To build the correlation model, the input signal is divided into two parts: a training part $\mathcal{T} = \{1,\ldots,m\}$ and an evaluation part $\mathcal{E} = \{m+1,\ldots,N\}$. On the training part, we select points $\mathcal{M} = \{n_1,\ldots,n_M\} \subseteq \mathcal{T}$ representative of the breathing pattern (i.e., points at maximum inspiration and expiration as well as points halfway between). Now let $L_{i,j,n}$ be the time series of the IR LEDs (i is the number of the LED, $j = 1,\ldots,3$ are the spatial coordinates, and n is the temporal index) and let $F_{k,j,n}$ be the time series of the gold fiducials (k is the fiducial number, j and n as before).

We will also make use of PCA to reduce the dimensionality of the LEDs' positions to one. In this case, $\tilde{L}_{i,\cdot,n}$ denotes the n-th sample of the principal component of the point cloud $L_{i,\cdot}$.

All correlation methods are based on one general assumption: there is a function f which we can use to compute the position and orientation of the target region based on information acquired on the patient's chest or abdomen. It is clear that, although some kind of function is bound to exist, the correlation between chest wall motion and interior organ motion cannot be expected to be completely deterministic. Even if we regard the body as a system of interacting elastic and inelastic tissues, we will not be able to perfectly model the correlation function for a single individual due to the complex nature of human motion.

5.1.1 Polynomial Correlation

The easiest approach to compute the correlation function f is to place radiopaque fiducials inside the target region and to attach markers to the patient's chest. Using a tracking system and biplanar fluoroscopy, the correlation between fiducial and marker motion can be determined. Subsequently, a polynomial model can be fitted to compute the position vector $F_{k,\cdot,n}$ of fiducial k from the position vector $L_{i,\cdot,n}$ of LED i, i.e.,

$$F_{k,\cdot,n} = f(L_{i,\cdot,n}),$$

where $f : \mathbb{R}^3 \mapsto \mathbb{R}^3$ is a polynomial of arbitrary degree. Since first experiments had shown that motion on the chest is predominantly along one axis (perpendicular to the chest wall), the initial simple correlation model was reduced to a polynomial $f : \mathbb{R} \mapsto \mathbb{R}^3$, i.e., the polynomial now reads

$$F_{k,\cdot,n} = f(\tilde{L}_{i,\cdot,n}).$$

Consequently, using the training set $\mathcal{M} = \{n_1, \ldots, n_M\}$, we can compute the coefficients of f as the least squares solution of a system of linear equations:

$$
V_i \begin{pmatrix} c_{0,1} & c_{0,2} & c_{0,3} \\ c_{1,1} & c_{1,2} & c_{1,3} \\ & \vdots & \\ c_{n,1} & c_{n,2} & c_{n,3} \end{pmatrix} = \begin{pmatrix} \mathbf{F}_{k,1,n_1} & \mathbf{F}_{k,2,n_1} & \mathbf{F}_{k,3,n_1} \\ \mathbf{F}_{k,1,n_2} & \mathbf{F}_{k,2,n_2} & \mathbf{F}_{k,3,n_2} \\ & \vdots & \\ \mathbf{F}_{k,1,n_M} & \mathbf{F}_{k,2,n_M} & \mathbf{F}_{k,3,n_M} \end{pmatrix}
$$

Here, n is the degree of the polynomial and V_i is the $M \times n$-Vandermode matrix of the point cloud $\{\tilde{\mathbf{L}}_{i,\cdot,n}\}_{n \in \mathcal{M}}$:

$$
V_i = \begin{pmatrix} 1 & \tilde{\mathbf{L}}_{i,\cdot,n_1} & \left(\tilde{\mathbf{L}}_{i,\cdot,n_1}\right)^2 & \cdots & \left(\tilde{\mathbf{L}}_{i,\cdot,n_1}\right)^n \\ 1 & \tilde{\mathbf{L}}_{i,\cdot,n_2} & \left(\tilde{\mathbf{L}}_{i,\cdot,n_2}\right)^2 & \cdots & \left(\tilde{\mathbf{L}}_{i,\cdot,n_2}\right)^n \\ \vdots & \vdots & \vdots & \cdots & \vdots \\ 1 & \tilde{\mathbf{L}}_{i,\cdot,n_M} & \left(\tilde{\mathbf{L}}_{i,\cdot,n_M}\right)^2 & \cdots & \left(\tilde{\mathbf{L}}_{i,\cdot,n_M}\right)^n \end{pmatrix}
$$

One problem of respiratory motion, however, is the fact that it exhibits hysteresis: assume that a point p moves from p_{ex} to p_{in} during one respiratory cycle. Hysteresis means that the path $p_{ex} \rightsquigarrow p_{in}$ is not the same as the path $p_{in} \rightsquigarrow p_{ex}$. This behaviour is due to differences in volume-to-pressure ratios during inspiration and expiration [40]. The polynomial model is able to capture this hysteresis if it is modified to use two polynomials, one for inspiration and one for expiration, i.e., the training set $\mathcal{M}$ is split into two sets, $\mathcal{M}_{in}$ and $\mathcal{M}_{ex}$ and two functions f_{in} and f_{ex} are built. We will call this model *dual polynomial*. $\mathcal{M}$ is split into the inhalation and exhalation parts by using a threshold speed v_t:

$$
n \in \mathcal{M} \Rightarrow v_n := \frac{\tilde{\mathbf{L}}_{i,\cdot,n+1} - \tilde{\mathbf{L}}_{i,\cdot,n-1}}{2\Delta t} \Rightarrow \begin{cases} n \curvearrowright \mathcal{M}_{in} & \text{if } v_n \geq -v_t \\ n \curvearrowright \mathcal{M}_{ex} & \text{if } v_n \leq v_t \end{cases}
$$

Here, Δt is the sampling rate of the signal. Using this splitting method, samples with slow speed will be placed in both $\mathcal{M}_{in}$ and $\mathcal{M}_{ex}$ to ensure that both end-inspiration and end-expiration are modelled by both flanks of the hysteresis. Nevertheless, a severe limitation of the initial (dual) polynomial models is the fact that they are built using sparse training data: in clinical settings, the patient is placed on the treatment couch and five to twelve data points are used to create the model. It is clear that, using this few samples, it is nearly impossible to cover the patient's complete breathing cycle. Furthermore, since respiratory amplitudes change over time, it is reasonable to assume that measurements outside the data recorded for training will occur, resulting in possibly high errors, especially for higher order polynomials. Due to this reason, a fallback mechanism is implemented: in addition to the inspiration and expiration polynomials, a linear function f_{lin} is fitted to all of $\mathcal{M}$ and is used for correlation whenever measurements outside the range of the training data occur, i.e., whenever

$$
\tilde{\mathbf{L}}_{i,\cdot,n} \notin \mathfrak{R} := \left[\min_{m \in \mathcal{M}} \left(\tilde{\mathbf{L}}_{i,\cdot,m}\right), \max_{m \in \mathcal{M}} \left(\tilde{\mathbf{L}}_{i,\cdot,m}\right) \right].
$$

Using this approach, however, does not ensure that the transition between the higher-order polynomial branches of the model to the linear model is smooth. This can be overcome by incorporating a blending mechanism. Let

$$r_1 = \min \mathfrak{R}, \quad r_2 = \max \mathfrak{R}, \quad r_3 = \sigma \left(r_2 - r_1 \right)$$

and let

$$\mathfrak{R}^- = [r_1 + 2r_3, r_2 - 2r_3]$$
$$\mathfrak{R}_1^{\leftarrow} = [r_1 + r_3, r_1 + 2r_3], \quad \mathfrak{R}_1^{\rightarrow} = [r_2 - 2r_3, r_2 - r_3]$$
$$\mathfrak{R}_2^{\leftarrow} = [r_1 - r_3, r_1 + r_3], \quad \mathfrak{R}_2^{\rightarrow} = [r_2 - r_3, r_2 + r_3]$$
$$\mathfrak{R}^+ = \mathfrak{R}_2^{\leftarrow} \cup \mathfrak{R}_1^{\leftarrow} \cup \mathfrak{R}^- \cup \mathfrak{R}_1^{\rightarrow} \cup \mathfrak{R}_2^{\rightarrow}.$$

Here, σ is a parameter determining the amount of overlap. A reasonable value would be $\sigma = 0.05$. These ranges are illustrated in figure 5.1. Then let

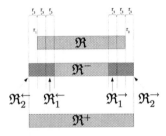

Fig. 5.1: Ranges for blending the polynomial model

$$d_{x,1}^{\leftarrow} = \frac{x - r_1 - 2r_3}{2r_3}, \quad d_{x,1}^{\rightarrow} = \frac{x - r_2 + 2r_3}{2r_3},$$
$$d_{x,2}^{\leftarrow} = \frac{x - r_1 - r_3}{r_3}, \quad d_{x,2}^{\rightarrow} = \frac{x - r_2 + r_3}{r_3}.$$

If we now also split the evaluation set $\mathscr{E}$ into an inhalation part $\mathscr{E}_{in}$ and an exhalation part $\mathscr{E}_{ex}$, we can finally specify the complete dual polynomial correlation algorithm:

$$f(x) = \begin{cases} f_{in}(x) & \text{if } x \in \mathfrak{R}^- \cap \mathscr{E}_{in} \\ f_{ex}(x) & \text{if } x \in \mathfrak{R}^- \cap \mathscr{E}_{ex} \\ \left(1 - d_{x,1}^{\rightarrow}\right) f_{in}(x) + d_{x,1}^{\rightarrow} \tfrac{1}{2} \left(f_{in}(x) + f_{ex}(x)\right) & \text{if } x \in \mathfrak{R}_1^{\rightarrow} \cap \mathscr{E}_{in} \\ \left(1 - d_{x,1}^{\rightarrow}\right) f_{ex}(x) + d_{x,1}^{\rightarrow} \tfrac{1}{2} \left(f_{in}(x) + f_{ex}(x)\right) & \text{if } x \in \mathfrak{R}_1^{\rightarrow} \cap \mathscr{E}_{ex} \\ \left(1 - d_{x,1}^{\leftarrow}\right) f_{in}(x) + d_{x,1}^{\leftarrow} \tfrac{1}{2} \left(f_{in}(x) + f_{ex}(x)\right) & \text{if } x \in \mathfrak{R}_1^{\leftarrow} \cap \mathscr{E}_{in} \\ \left(1 - d_{x,1}^{\leftarrow}\right) f_{ex}(x) + d_{x,1}^{\leftarrow} \tfrac{1}{2} \left(f_{in}(x) + f_{ex}(x)\right) & \text{if } x \in \mathfrak{R}_1^{\leftarrow} \cap \mathscr{E}_{ex} \\ \left(1 - d_{x,2}^{\leftarrow}\right) \tfrac{1}{2} \left(f_{in}(x) + f_{ex}(x)\right) + d_{x,2}^{\leftarrow} f_{ex}(x) & \text{if } x \in \mathfrak{R}_2^{\leftarrow} \\ \left(1 - d_{x,2}^{\rightarrow}\right) \tfrac{1}{2} \left(f_{in}(x) + f_{ex}(x)\right) + d_{x,2}^{\rightarrow} f_{ex}(x) & \text{if } x \in \mathfrak{R}_2^{\rightarrow} \\ f_{lin}(x) & \text{if } x \notin \mathfrak{R}^+ \end{cases}$$

Note that, in contrast to $\mathscr{M}_{in}$ and $\mathscr{M}_{ex}$, the sets $\mathscr{E}_{in}$ and $\mathscr{E}_{ex}$ must not overlap. This can be achieved by using a thresholded search for extremal values instead of the velocity threshold. This can be done according to the algorithm shown in listing E.3 in appendix E.

Example 14. Let x be a simulated respiratory signal (see appendix D) using $A = 2$, $f = 0.25$, $e_1 = 8$, $e_2 = 4$ and $t = (0, 0.01, \ldots, 100)^T$. The modification parameters were $\delta_A = 0.1$, $\delta_b = 0.05$, $\delta_B = 0.1$, $N_B = 10$, $\delta_T = 0.1$, $\sigma = 0.015$. Now the following correlation function is used:

$$f(x) = \frac{1}{2} \left(D(x, 30) + x\right) + \frac{1}{20} x^2 + \frac{2}{10} (x - 0.8)^3$$

This correlation function has a delay term, $D(x, 30)$, which creates a phase shift of 0.3 seconds between the internal and the external signal. It also has linear, quadratic and cubic terms. Using this model, the simulated internal signal y_n can be computed for $n = 1, \ldots, N - 30$. Here, $N = 10,001$, the number of samples in x. The signals x_n and $y_n = f(x_n)$ and their correlation plot are shown in figure 5.2.

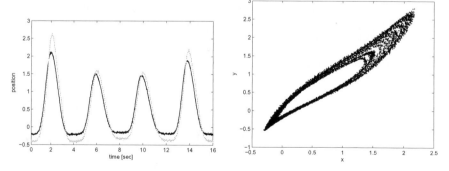

Fig. 5.2: Left: simulated respiratory signal x (black) and simulated internal signal $y = f(x)$ (grey). Right: correlation between the signals x and $y = f(x)$ as explained in example 14. Hysteresis and nonlinear correlation are clearly visible.

Using x and y, we now try to recover the correlation function f. The correlation models are built using thirteen samples (covering the first three cycles using one sample at maximum expiration, one at maximum inspiration and one halfway inbetween). To further clarify the blending method used, refer to figure 5.3. The resulting, recovered correlation functions are shown in figure 5.4.

From this figure, and from table 5.1, we can see that no single algorithm is clearly superior to all others and that they all suffer from considerable errors. What is clear, however, is that the dual polynomial models outperform the single models in all measures. Even more, if one algorithm should be selected, it would probably be the blended dual quadratic model: it has the lowest CI-0.95 and FC^{III}-0.30 values, i.e., its errors are the least periodic and the upper bound for 95 % of the samples is lowest.

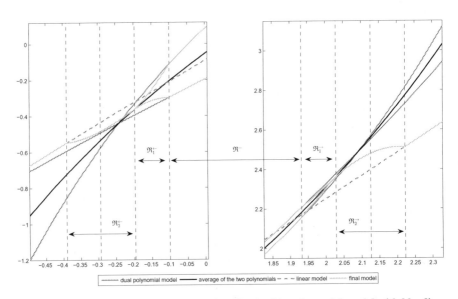

Fig. 5.3: Close-up of the blending mechanism. Dual cubic polynomial model with blending, see figure 5.4k. In $\mathfrak{R}^-$, the dual polynomial model (dark grey) is used. In $\mathfrak{R}_1$, the two branches of the dual polynomial model (dark grey) are blended to their average (black). In $\mathfrak{R}_2$, this average (black) is blended to the linear model (dashed grey). Outside $\mathfrak{R}^+ = \mathfrak{R}^- \cup \mathfrak{R}_1 \cup \mathfrak{R}_2$, the linear model (dashed grey) is used. The model which is finally used is overlayed in light grey.

5.1.2 Correlation with Support Vector Regression

The shortcomings of the polynomial correlation methods motivate the introduction of a new correlation model. This model is based on ε-SVR (for more details about

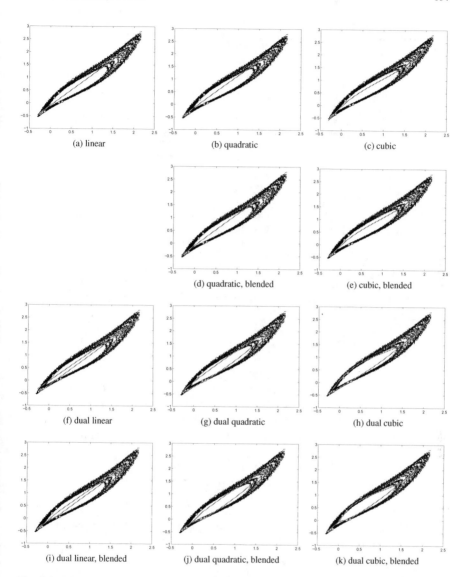

Fig. 5.4: Correlation functions computed by the polynomial algorithms. The black dots are the actual correlation, the grey curves are the computed functions and the light grey dots are the training samples.

Table 5.1: Errors of the polynomial correlation algorithms. Optimal results for each group (minimal RMS, CI, FC^{III}, and $\mathfrak{J}$) are shown in bold, globally optimal results are shown in bold italics.

degree	RMS	CI-0.50	CI-0.75	CI-0.95	FC^{III}-0.10	FC^{III}-0.30	$\mathfrak{J}$ [a]
single polynomial model							
linear	0.1997	**0.1102**	0.2451	0.3956	**0.1396**	**0.1396**	2.4121
quadratic	0.2006	0.1111	**0.2371**	0.4198	0.1396	0.1396	2.4620
cubic	**0.1901**	0.1235	0.2451	**0.3611**	0.1396	0.1396	2.8645
single polynomial model, blended [b]							
linear	—	—	—	—	—	—	—
quadratic	0.2007	**0.1101**	**0.2362**	0.4198	**0.1365**	**0.1365**	2.4338
cubic	**0.1905**	0.1231	0.2454	**0.3611**	0.1535	0.1535	2.6554
dual polynomial model							
linear	0.1666	0.1032	0.1997	0.3352	0.1590	0.1590	2.4281
quadratic	*0.1315*	0.0740	0.1487	*0.2741*	0.1291	*0.1291*	*2.3327*
cubic	0.1344	*0.0481*	*0.1234*	0.3130	*0.0721*	0.1890	2.7191
dual polynomial model, blended							
linear	0.1704	0.0911	0.2080	0.3373	0.1185	0.1185	2.3977
quadratic	**0.1363**	0.0796	0.1626	*0.2706*	0.0856	*0.0856*	**2.3719**
cubic	0.1363	**0.0614**	**0.1339**	0.3063	**0.0800**	0.1373	2.6136

---

[a] The original signal's jitter $\mathfrak{J}(y)$ is 2.2612.

[b] Blending makes no sense for the single linear model.

SVR, refer to section 4.2.4 and section A.2). In this model, we do not only use the LEDs' principal component of motion, as is done for the the polynomial models, but all three dimensions. Second, information about the direction of breathing is directly built into the model by creating vectors $\mathbf{D}_i$ indicating the direction of breathing:

$$\mathbf{D}_{i,n} = \begin{cases} -1 & \text{for } \tilde{\mathbf{L}}_{i,\cdot,n} - \tilde{\mathbf{L}}_{i,\cdot,n-1} < -v_t \\ 0 & \text{for } -v_t \leq \tilde{\mathbf{L}}_{i,\cdot,n} - \tilde{\mathbf{L}}_{i,\cdot,n-1} \leq v_t \;, \quad n = 2,\ldots,N. \\ 1 & \text{for } \tilde{\mathbf{L}}_{i,\cdot,n} - \tilde{\mathbf{L}}_{i,\cdot,n-1} > v_t \end{cases}$$

Third, information about, e.g., the signal's speed and acceleration are also incorporated by bringing in derivatives $\mathbf{L}^{(n)}$ of the LEDs' positions. These derivatives are computed using central differences, i.e.,

$$\mathbf{L}^{(n)}_{i,j,k} = \frac{\mathbf{L}^{(n-1)}_{i,j,k+1} - \mathbf{L}^{(n-1)}_{i,j,k-1}}{2\Delta t}.$$

Here, Δt is the temporal spacing of the signal. Now let

$$\mathbf{x}_{i,m} = \left(\mathbf{L}^{\mathrm{T}}_{i,\cdot,m}, {\mathbf{L}^{(1)}_{i,\cdot,m}}^{\mathrm{T}}, \ldots, {\mathbf{L}^{(n)}_{i,\cdot,m}}^{\mathrm{T}}, \mathbf{D}_{i,m} \right)^{\mathrm{T}} \in \mathbb{R}^{3+3\cdot n} \times \{-1,0,1\}.$$

Then for each i, j, and $m \in \mathcal{M}$ we create training samples

$$s_m^{i,j} = \left\{ \mathbf{x}_{i,m}, \tilde{\mathbf{F}}_{j,\cdot,m} \right\},$$

i.e., the samples $s_m^{i,j}, m \in \mathcal{M}$, describe the relation between LED i and $\tilde{\mathbf{F}}_{j,\cdot}$, the principal component of motion of fiducial j. These samples are then used to train ε-SVR machines which in turn serve as correlation models.

Example 15. We return to example 14. The SVR correlation models are now built using the same training samples as the polynomial models. Additionally, the first three derivatives are computed using central differences.

Then the SVR machines are trained using linear, polynomial or Gaussian RBF kernel functions (for explanation of the kernels, refer to section A.2, especially the subsection 'Kernel functions'). Since the SVR training has several parameters (ε, C, σ for linear, polynomial and Gaussian RBF kernels, τ and n for polynomial kernels), the models generated were optimised using a steepest descent method. The RMS value of the correlation served as objective which we sought to minimise. The resulting errors are given in table 5.2, the corresponding correlation graphs are shown in figure 5.5. In this case, the optimal algorithm in terms of RMS and CI uses two derivatives and a linear kernel. Its FC values are not optimal, but still the second-lowest. Its jitter, however, is relatively high: nearly double the original signal's value. If this is a concern, i.e., if the correlated signal should be as smooth as possible, the next choice would be to use one derivative and the Gaussian RBF kernel. Its jitter is even lower than the original signal's jitter, but the other measures are higher. The difficulty to find a proper trade-off between the different error measures now becomes obvious.

5.2 Experimental Validation

The correlation algorithms were validated using experimentally acquired data. Two studies were performed: first, the correlation between chest markers and implanted fiducials was evaluated in an animal study. Second, 3D US was used to track vessel bifurcations in the liver of volunteers.

5.2.1 Animal Study

For this work, four gold fiducials were implanted into the liver of a living swine under US guidance. Respiratory motion of the liver was recorded in two sessions while the swine was ventilated manually using a bag valve mask. The swine was killed minutes prior to the experiment. The experiment was performed in the context of the FUSION project, a part of the BMBF's SOMIT research focus.

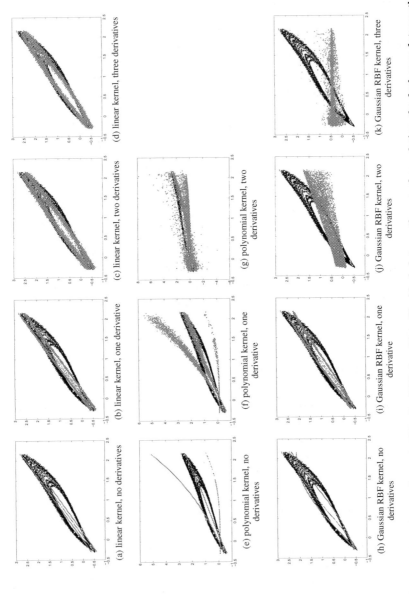

Fig. 5.5: Correlation functions as determined by the SVR algorithm. The black dots are the actual correlation, the dark grey dots are the output of the computed correlation models and the light grey dots are the training samples.

Table 5.2: Errors of the SVR correlation algorithms. Optimal results for each kernel function (minimal RMS, CI, and FC^{III}) are shown in bold, globally optimal results are shown in bold italics.

# of deriv.	RMS	CI-0.50	CI-0.75	CI-0.95	FC^{III}-0.10	FC^{III}-0.30	$\mathfrak{J}$ [a]
linear kernel function							
none	0.1567	0.1054	0.1547	0.3446	0.0667	0.0667	2.6242
one	0.1510	0.1072	0.1495	0.3226	0.0646	0.1123	**2.2294**
two	0.1158	0.0833	0.1374	0.2203	**0.0246**	*0.0246*	6.4057
three	*0.0929*	*0.0676*	*0.1093*	*0.1770*	0.0298	0.0298	4.4732
polynomial kernel function, degree two [b]							
none	**0.1830**	**0.1187**	**0.2379**	**0.3374**	0.0647	0.0647	**2.3356**
one	0.2996	0.1997	0.3441	0.5892	0.0215	**0.0544**	16.3073
two	0.2928	0.1919	0.3394	0.5662	*0.0174*	0.0857	16.4108
three	—	—	—	—	—	—	—
polynomial kernel function, degree three [b]							
none	**0.4800**	**0.1104**	**0.2375**	1.3030	**0.0687**	0.1752	**4.3195**
one	0.5487	0.1226	0.2912	1.4425	0.1163	0.1163	7.8432
two	0.6299	0.3173	0.5726	1.4477	0.0915	**0.1071**	37.5571
three	—	—	—	—	—	—	—
Gaussian RBF kernel function							
none	0.1351	**0.0796**	**0.1218**	0.2981	0.0764	0.1437	2.4300
one	**0.1339**	0.0851	0.1568	**0.2694**	**0.0449**	0.1166	*2.0322*
two	0.5357	0.3968	0.5705	1.0479	0.0812	0.1412	19.5301
three	0.8797	0.7224	0.9062	1.7275	0.1119	**0.1119**	8.6305

[a] The original signal's jitter $\mathfrak{J}(y)$ is 2.2612.
[b] It was not possible to optimise the SVR correlation model for three derivatives.

5.2.1.1 Setup

To acquire the fiducials' 3D position, a two-plane X-ray imaging device (Philips Allura Xper FD20/10$^{(O)}$, figure 5.6a) at the Institute for Neuroradiology (University Hospital Schleswig-Holstein, Lübeck) was used. It can take X-ray shots with a resolution of 1024x1024 pixels at a frame rate of up to 15 Hz.

To record the swine's chest surface motion, a net of 19 IR LEDs (see [18] and figure 5.6b) was placed on the swine's abdomen. The LEDs were tracked using the Atracsys accuTrack 250 system, effectively delivering a recording frame rate of 216 Hz for each LED. The signals were then downsampled to 15 Hz to match the acquisition speed of the X-ray cameras.

To determine the geometric relation between the two X-ray imaging units and the tracking camera, a custom calibration rig (see figure 5.7) was used: an acrylic box (10x7x5 cm^3) with twelve embedded metallic spheres and eight LEDs was built. The system was calibrated by simultaneously acquiring an image of the calibration rig with the X-ray devices and determining the rig's position using the tracking camera. The actual calibration was performed using the POSIT algorithm [5], resulting in a projection error of less than one pixel (RMS). Both the LEDs and the metal spheres could be detected with sub-millimetre accuracy.

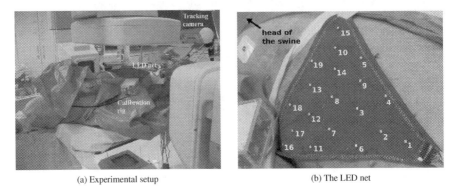

(a) Experimental setup   (b) The LED net

Fig. 5.6: X-ray device, tracking camera, calibration rig and LED net

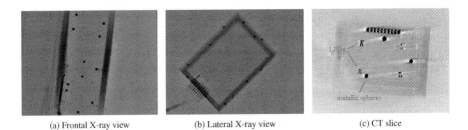

(a) Frontal X-ray view   (b) Lateral X-ray view   (c) CT slice

Fig. 5.7: The calibration rig

The frame grabber and the IR tracking system are connected to one machine (Intel Q9450, 8 GiB RAM, CentOS 5 x64).

5.2.1.2 Recording fluoroscopic video

Since the X-ray system does not allow real-time recording of image sequences of arbitrary length, a high resolution/high speed frame grabbing system (Matrox Helios XA$^{(P)}$) was used. The X-ray device outputs images at a frame rate of up to 15 Hz which are not directly available for recording. We thus attached the frame grabbing card to the video lines used to display the X-ray images in the examination room. These video lines output an 8 bit grey scale signal with a resolution of 1280x1024 pixels at a frame rate of 76 Hz. The resulting acquisition data rate of $2 \cdot 76 \cdot 1280 \cdot 1024 = 199,229,440$ bytes per second (i.e., 190 MB/sec) cannot be written to disk in real time, not even to the RAID hard disk array used. But since not all images need to be recorded, a filtering algorithm can be employed to detect when a new X-ray shot was taken. Let A_i be the last available image and let A_{i+1} be the image which has just been acquired by the frame grabber. Then the standard deviation of the difference image $A_{i+1} - A_i$ was computed and a threshold τ was selected such that $\mathrm{std}\,(A_{i+1} - A_i) < \tau$ for all grabbed images A_i and A_{i+1} which come from the same X-ray shot. Figure 5.8 shows the histogram of these standard deviations for a recording session of 60,765 images (corresponding to 13:19.5 minutes). This

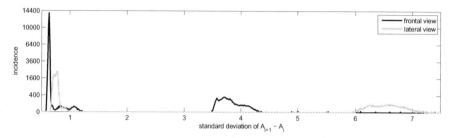

Fig. 5.8: Histogram of the standard deviation of successive image differences for the frontal (black) and lateral (grey) acquisition devices. Note the quadratic scaling along the y-axis.

figure clearly shows that there is a gap in the distribution for both acquisition channels. The first peak (standard deviation of approximately 0.6 to 1.3) corresponds to acquisition and processing noise while the second peak (3.5 to 4.4 for the frontal view and 6.0 to 7.3 for the lateral view) corresponds to motion in the image and X-ray noise. Selecting a threshold of $\tau = 3$ resulted in very good separation of the images. Using this thresholding and by only saving the 1000x1000 pixel region actually showing X-ray data, the data rate can be reduced to 28.6 MB/sec. This can be further reduced to 6.5 MB/sec by using moderate JPEG compression[2]. The recording software also features video recording of uncompressed or MJPEG video data at 15 Hz, corresponding to an average data rate of 28.6 and 1.6 MB/sec, respectively. The recording GUI is shown in figure 5.9.

5.2.1.3 Tracking the gold fiducials

To track the gold fiducials in the X-ray images, a graphical tool kit written in C++ to perform Region of Interest (ROI) based segmentation of ellipsoidal objects and triangulate the 3D position of the fiducials was developed (figures 5.10 to 5.13). Using this GUI, it is possible to enter the current intrinsic parameters of the X-ray camera system (figure 5.10a). Furthermore, it can be used to detect the lead balls of a calibration phantom (figure 5.10b and figure 5.11), to compute the extrinsic parameters of the camera system (figure 5.10c) and to perform triangulation with respect to a second tracking modality. Figure 5.12 shows the typical application of the calibrated tracking software: the two views of the test subject are shown, one fiducial is selected in both planes (using interactive ROI placement) and the triangulated position is shown. Using the tracking software, it is possible to automatically

---

[2] The quantisation factor $Q \in [0, 99]$ was set to 10. Higher values correspond to stronger compression.

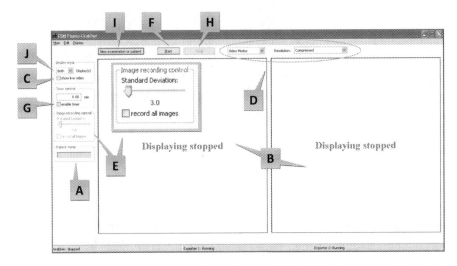

Fig. 5.9: GUI of the fluoroscopic recording software. The indivdual parts are: (A) patient name, (B) video panels, (C) check box to show/hide live video, (D) recording mode selector, (E) filtering algorithm, (F) start button, (G) recording timer, (H) stop button, (I) new examination/ patient button, (J) view selection box.

advance through the recorded image and adjust the position of the ROIs to account for motion.

Segmentation is done in multiple steps: for each ROI, a detailed view (figure 5.13) can be shown. First, the image can be smoothed using pyramid up-/downsampling, median filtering or Gaussian filtering. The image can also be eroded and dilated to remove artefacts. Second, an edge detector (Canny or Sobel) can be applied to find the contours present in the image. Third, very small contours, i.e., below a certain user-defined threshold, are discarded and only the remaining closed contours are reported. These settings can be adjusted as shown in figure 5.10b.

As additional information, four moments of the contours are computed: its orientation Θ, i.e., the angle of the largest eigenvector, its eigenvalues λ_1 and λ_2, i.e., the lengths of the contour's semiaxes, and the contour's eccentricity.

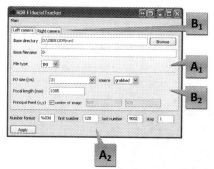

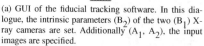

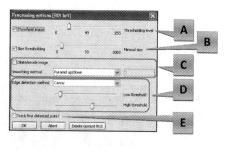

(a) GUI of the fiducial tracking software. In this dialogue, the intrinsic parameters (B_2) of the two (B_1) X-ray cameras are set. Additionally (A_1, A_2), the input images are specified.

(b) Parameter selection for fiducial segmentation. The figure shows the thresholding settings (A), the minimal size a detected contour must have (B), image smoothing settings (C), edge detector settings (D), and whether the ROI should try to follow a detected point.

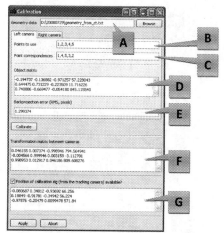

(c) Calibration dialogue. Here, the geometry data file can be selected (A), the points from the geometry file which will be used for calibration are entered (B), the correspondence to the numbers from the ROI is entered (C, see also figure 5.11), the computed pose of the calibration phantom is shown (D), the RMS backprojection error is shown (E), the transform matrix between the two cameras is given (F) and, optionally, the pose of the rig with respect to a second tracking modality can be entered (G).

Fig. 5.10: Settings dialogues of the fiducial tracking software.

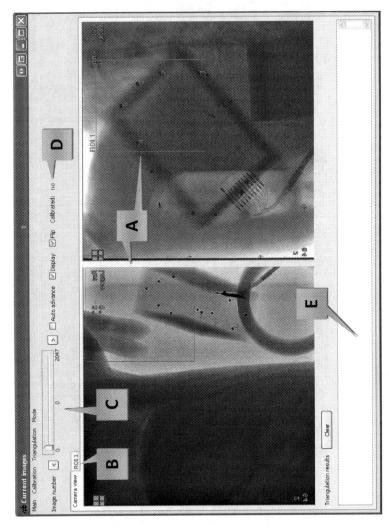

Fig. 5.11: Main window of the fiducial tracking software. This view shows the ROIs used for calibration (A), the tab to switch to the detailed ROI view (B), the display control (C), the calibration status (D) and the triangulation output (E). Note that, in all ROIs, the detected fiducials are marked with red numbers. The calibration rig and the animal subject are clearly visible.

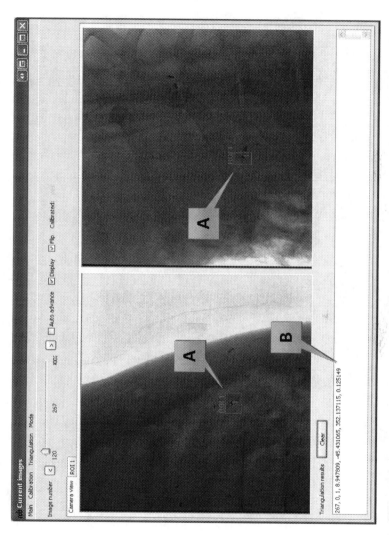

Fig. 5.12: View of the GUI used for the animal experiment. Here, one fiducial is selected (A) and its triangulation results are shown (B). The text box shows the image number, a status flag, the point number, the point's x, y, and z coordinates and the triangulation error. Both the fiducials and the LEDs are clearly visible.

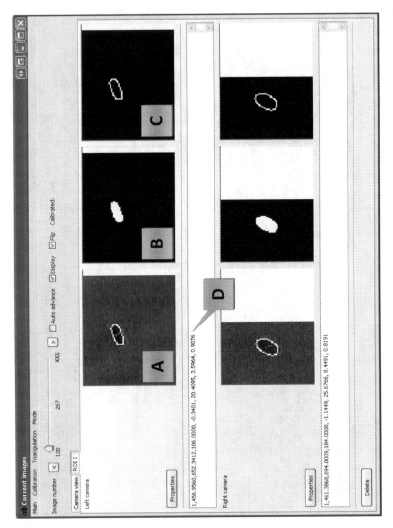

Fig. 5.13: Detailed view of one ROI. Here, the original image (A) with superimposed contours (white) and tracked centre of gravity (red), the smoothed and thresholded image (B), the detected contours (C) and contour statistics (D) are shown. The statistics are the ROI number, the point's x and y coordinates, the contour's size, its orientation (Θ), its eigenvalues (λ_1 and λ_2) and its eccentricity.

5.2.1.4 Results

To validate the algorithms, two datasets were recorded. The first one has a length of 2:09.94 minutes, the second one is 9:52.16 minutes long. Only LEDs 11, 14, and 16 to 19 were visible during the first recording. During the second recording, however, LEDs 6 to 14 and 16 to 19 were visible. In both cases, all four fiducials could be tracked. Figure 5.14 shows the spatial relation of the LEDs and fiducials in both test runs. LEDs which are adjacent on the net (see figure 5.6b) are connected with red lines.

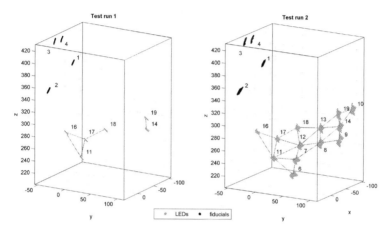

Fig. 5.14: 3D overview of the recordings done. LEDs are shown in grey, fiducials are shown in black and the red lines show adjacent LEDs on the LED net.

Analysis of LED motion shows that it is not only in one direction and does exhibit strong hysteresis relative to fiducial motion. This is the first indication that the simple polynomial models are not adequate.

Evaluation results for the best polynomial model (biquadratic with blending) and for the ε-SVR model are given in figure 5.15. The polynomial model does not only incur a larger RMS error (see table 5.3) but also suffers from periodic errors at the inspiration and expiration peaks. Figure 5.16 shows the second signal.

The correlation plots of all the polynomial correlation models are given in figure 5.17. Ideally, the grey curves would cover all black dots. Clearly, the simple polynomial models don't fit the data very well, the bipolynomial models' matching is better. The actual numbers are given in table 5.3. The reason for the high periodic error of the polynomial model is that it does not adequately capture correlation at end-inspiration and end-expiration. These regions are marked with black dotted rectangles in figure 5.17k.

Evaluation of the ε-SVR correlation model shows a much better matching: figure 5.18 shows the correlation plots of the SVR correlation model using a linear kernel function (top), polynomial kernel function (centre) and RBF kernel function

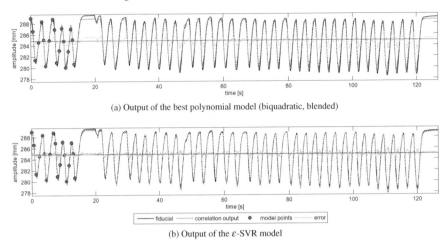

(a) Output of the best polynomial model (biquadratic, blended)

(b) Output of the ε-SVR model

Fig. 5.15: First test run, results of the correlation process. First 60 s are shown. Fiducial motion is shown in black, training points used with black circles and the correlation output in dark grey. The residual error is plotted in light grey. The respiratory pause around $t = 20$ s is accidental and not connected to the correlation model.

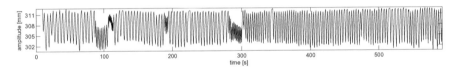

Fig. 5.16: Second test run. The signal shows variations in breathing frequency and amplitude.

(bottom). In all cases, optimal parameters were selected and the prinicipal components of LED eleven's motion versus the principal component of fiducial one are plotted. Clearly, the grey dots (output of the correlation model) correspond very well to the black dots (actual correlation). This is also reflected in the numbers given in table 5.3: the SVR approach outperforms the best (bi)polynomial model by 67 % (signal 1) or 66 % (signal 2). Furthermore, the SVR model does not suffer as much from systematic errors like the polynomial models do.

5.2.1.5 Selection of LEDs and using multiple LEDs

Since one reason to investigate the SVR correlation model was the possibility to easily increase dimensionality of the input data, the model was also evalutated for selecting different and/or multiple surrogate LEDs. Two experiments were performed:

1. The SVR model was built using the parameters from the optimisation for the first LED.

Table 5.3: Errors of the correlation algorithms, porcine study. Optimal results for each group (minimal RMS, CI, FC^III, and ℑ) are shown in bold, globally optimal results are shown in bold italics.

(a) First test run

Errors of the different polynomial correlation algorithms

degree	RMS	CI-0.50	CI-0.75	CI-0.95	FC^III_-0.10	FC^III_-0.30	ℑ
single polynomial model							
linear	1.0557	0.7720	1.3245	1.9390	0.2084	0.2084	4.7341
quadratic	**1.0067**	0.7150	**1.3036**	**1.8315**	0.2032	0.2032	**4.7334**
cubic	1.0988	**0.5392**	1.4027	2.2669	**0.1432**	**0.1432**	5.3812
single polynomial model, blended							
linear	1.0165	0.7852	**1.2991**	**1.8315**	0.1980	0.1980	**4.7784**
cubic	1.0928	**0.5619**	1.3719	2.2582	**0.1514**	**0.1514**	4.8809
dual polynomial model							
linear	0.8703	0.6991	1.0719	1.6510	0.1459	0.1459	**5.1846**
quadratic	**0.6420**	**0.3334**	**0.6012**	**1.3527**	0.0982	0.0982	5.2002
cubic	0.7056	0.3655	0.7062	1.4676	**0.0893**	**0.0893**	5.4369
dual polynomial model, blended							
linear	0.8534	0.5979	0.9919	1.6510	0.1842	0.1842	**4.8170**
quadratic	**0.6268**	0.3613	**0.6026**	**1.2081**	0.1258	0.1258	4.8543
cubic	0.6824	**0.3310**	0.7027	1.4035	**0.1171**	**0.1171**	4.8873

Errors of the SVR correlation algorithms

# of deriv.	RMS	CI-0.50	CI-0.75	CI-0.95	FC^III_-0.10	FC^III_-0.30	ℑ
linear kernel function							
none	0.4732	0.2821	0.5346	0.8990	0.1180	0.1180	6.2136
one	0.3313	0.2324	0.3734	0.6480	0.0731	0.1237	5.7245
two	0.2787	0.1440	0.2795	0.6111	0.0588	0.1022	5.9122
three	**0.2393**	**0.1198**	**0.2218**	**0.5224**	**0.0513**	**0.0883**	**5.5987**
polynomial kernel function, degree two							
none	74.1255	49.5472	86.5331	144.9357	0.1060	0.1885	371.2283
one	0.2919	*0.1123*	*0.1956*	0.6661	0.0687	0.0687	6.0640
two	**0.2562**	0.1412	0.2555	**0.5357**	**0.0612**	**0.0612**	5.7796
three	3.3414	0.3637	0.9772	3.8230	0.0804	0.2750	22.2263
Gaussian RBF kernel function							
none	0.3588	0.2043	0.3628	0.6215	0.0745	0.0745	***5.5943***
one	*0.2089*	*0.1281*	*0.2291*	*0.4181*	0.0465	0.1238	5.7070
two	0.4784	0.1841	0.3315	0.7392	*0.0357*	*0.0648*	6.3786
three	2.8611	2.0940	3.3605	5.4471	0.1174	0.1996	24.9952

(b) second test run

Errors of the different polynomial correlation algorithms

degree	RMS	CI-0.50	CI-0.75	CI-0.95	FC^III_-0.10	FC^III_-0.30	ℑ
single polynomial model							
linear	**1.0267**	**0.6806**	**1.2178**	**2.0105**	0.1487	0.1487	4.7814
quadratic	1.0316	0.6836	1.2195	2.0283	0.1479	0.1479	4.7774
cubic	1.1052	0.7953	1.3364	2.1184	*0.1130*	*0.1130*	**4.7099**
single polynomial model, blended							
linear	1.0319	**0.6872**	**1.2188**	**2.0283**	0.1481	0.1481	4.7796
cubic	1.0905	0.7664	1.3117	2.1159	0.1346	0.1346	*4.6305*
dual polynomial model							
linear	0.9843	**0.6597**	**1.1856**	1.9159	0.1580	0.1580	4.9529
quadratic	0.9732	0.6655	1.1965	**1.8722**	0.1589	0.1589	4.9220
cubic	1.0063	0.7212	1.2522	1.9226	0.1520	0.1520	4.9023
dual polynomial model, blended							
linear	0.9856	0.6541	1.1952	1.9159	0.1581	0.1581	4.8967
quadratic	*0.9703*	*0.6530*	1.1870	1.8722	0.1586	0.1586	4.8959
cubic	0.9962	0.7040	1.2219	1.9226	**0.1533**	**0.1533**	4.8399

Errors of the SVR correlation algorithms

# of deriv.	RMS	CI-0.50	CI-0.75	CI-0.95	FC^III_-0.10	FC^III_-0.30	ℑ
linear kernel function							
none	0.3531	0.2435	0.4098	0.6896	0.0448	0.0800	5.4527
one	*0.3276*	*0.2219*	*0.3809*	*0.6349*	0.0507	0.0901	5.1681
two	0.4627	0.2653	0.5106	0.8449	**0.0422**	**0.0791**	*4.9307*
three	0.8490	0.3851	0.7565	1.6622	0.0533	0.1392	5.8827
polynomial kernel function, degree two							
none	63.7179	43.0489	71.6391	123.7499	0.0732	0.1345	121.7536
one	0.4212	0.2607	0.4726	0.8661	0.0830	0.0830	**5.2842**
two	0.5992	0.2991	0.5640	1.0255	*0.0260*	*0.0451*	5.3755
three	50.8086	1.1229	2.8082	19.4670	0.1592	0.1592	134.5575
Gaussian RBF kernel function							
none	**0.7685**	**0.5354**	**0.9184**	**1.4984**	0.1255	0.1255	**4.9793**
one	0.7934	0.5666	0.9304	1.5427	0.0836	0.0836	5.1451
two	1.0165	0.6041	1.0819	1.8984	**0.0539**	0.0927	7.0304
three	2.7454	1.9036	3.2186	5.3380	0.0657	0.1905	24.9289

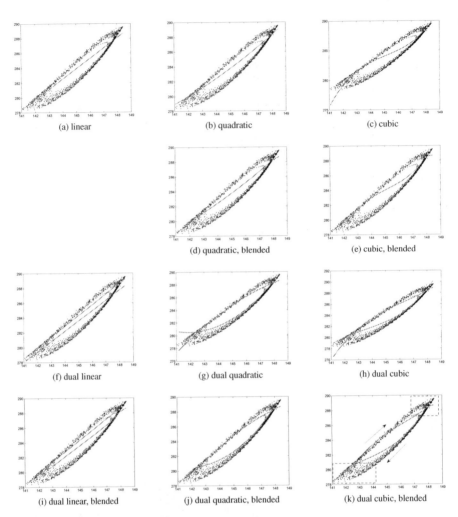

Fig. 5.17: Correlation functions computed by the polynomial algorithms for the first test run. The x-axis shows the principal component of the motion of LED 11, the y-axis shows the principal component of motion of the first fiducial. Model points are marked with grey circles, the model output is shown in grey. In (k), the dotted boxes show the areas corresponding to maximum inspiration and expiration; the arrows indicate the breathing direction.

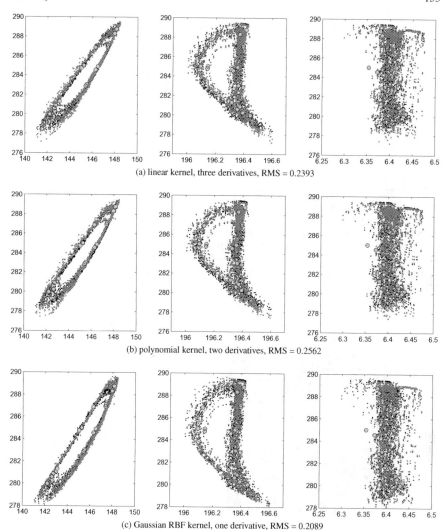

Fig. 5.18: The best ε-SVR models for the first test run. The x-axes show the motion of LED 11 (after PCA), the y-axes show the principal component of motion of the first fiducial. Model points are marked with grey circles, the model output is shown in grey.

2. The SVR model was built using optimised parameters for each LED or combination of LEDs.

We also investigated the influence of LED selection on the quality of the correlation model. When selecting different LEDs as input surrogates, we see that on the first signal, the RMS error ranges from 0.17 mm to 0.28 mm whereas on the second signal, it ranges from 0.25 mm to 2.67 mm. Since the ε-SVR correlation model has been designed such that it can use input from more than one LED at a time, we evaluated the model for all possible pairs (triplets, quadruplets, ...). The results are shown in figure 5.19 for the first signal and in figure 5.20 for the second signal.

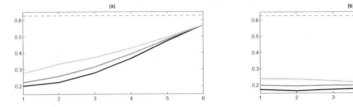

Fig. 5.19: The plots show the range (minimum and maximum values) and mean of the RMS error when using multiple LEDs on the first signal. (a) shows the resulting RMS error when the SVR machine is trained using the optimal parameters from table 5.3. (b) shows the results when the SVR machine's parameters are optimised for each LED set. Read: when using three LEDs (20 possibilites) to build the correlation model, the resulting RMS error is, depending on the selected triplet, between 0.28 and 0.37 mm with a mean of 0.32 mm when using the old parameters and between 0.17 and 0.23 mm with a mean of 0.20 mm when using optimal parameters.

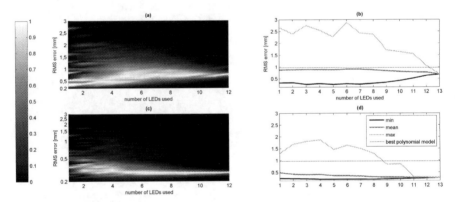

Fig. 5.20: Graphs (b) and (d) show the range (minimum and maximum values) and mean of the RMS error when using multiple LEDs on the second signal. (b) was computed with the parameters from table 5.3 and (d) was computed with optimal parameters for each LED set. Additionally, graphs (a) and (c) show the distribution of the RMS error. Note the logarithmic scale along the y-axis of graph (c).

We can see that on the first signal, using more than one LED does not noticeably improve correlation results, possibly due to overfitting. On the second signal, however, the best attainable correlation model uses eight LEDs and outperforms the best model using one LED by 15 %: the RMS value drops from 0.25 mm to 0.21 mm. In this case, the best polynomial model is outperformed by as much as 78 %. Additionally, the 95 % CI drops to 0.35 mm. We can clearly see that in this case the model using more LEDs is capable of catching the changing characteristics of the signal. Note that on signal one, only 19 and on signal two, only 17 samples are used to build the model which is evaluated on 1,876 and 8,588 samples, respectively.

5.2.2 Human Data[3]

Since the results from the porcine study are very promising, a second study with human volunteers was performed. In this study, the aim was to collect internal and external motion traces to further validate the proposed new correlation model. The method of choice for internal measurements, since fluoroscopy and fiducial implantation was not possible, was three-dimensional live US. External data was recorded in the same way as in the porcine study, using IR LEDs and the accuTrack 250 system.

To create external surrogates, a chest belt was used. It consists of a tight-fitting, elastic rubber band with 16 LEDs. US volumes were recorded using our GE Vivid7 Dimension station. The 3V 3D/4D transducer for cardiac imaging was used. The transducer was attached to an adept Viper s850 robot which in turn was tracked using a four-LED marker. Figure 5.22 shows the setup used.

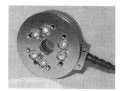

Fig. 5.21: ATI IA Mini45 6 DOF force-torque sensor

To simplify initial alignment and to keep up with possible movements of the volunteer, the robot is equipped with a Mini45 6 DOF force-torque sensor[(Q)]. This sensor, shown in figure 5.21, is mounted between the robot's endeffector and the US transducer. The sensor is calibrated using the method presented in [28]. With this calibration, the sensor only reports external forces applied to the tool attached and, using the robot's position and orientation information, automatically compensates for the forces and torques exerted by the tool.

The US station was modified by creating a code-upload function to execute image processing and tracking algorithms directly on the machine. This functionality eliminates the bottleneck of having to transfer the volumetric data to another computer for analysis.

5.2.2.1 Synchronisation

To calibrate the temporal offset between the US station's and the tracking camera's time stamps, we used a calibration phantom: a lead ball on a nylon wire is mounted in a plastic bracket which is moved by the robot in a water tank. The lead ball can be tracked easily using the US station and a maximum intensity search. Additionally, an LED is attached to the mounting post of the bracket. The phantom is shown in figure 5.23. Now a sinusoidal up-and-down motion with changing amplitude is

---

[3] Parts of this section have been published in [6, 7].

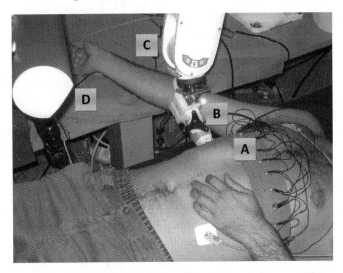

Fig. 5.22: Setup of the US data acquisition. (A) shows the chest belt with LEDs, (B) shows the US transducer with attached 4-LED-marker, (C) shows the robot guiding the transducer and (D) shows the tracking camera.

performed by the robot. The motion is $z(t) = A(t) \cdot \sin(2\pi t)$, where

$$A(t) = \begin{cases} t & \text{for } 0 \leq t < 10 \\ 20 - t & \text{for } 10 \leq t \leq 20 \end{cases}$$

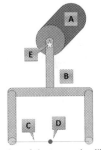

(a) Drawing of the temporal calibration phantom. (A) is the robot's endeffector, (B) is the plastic phantom, (C) is the nylon wire, (D) is the lead ball and (E) is the tracking LED.

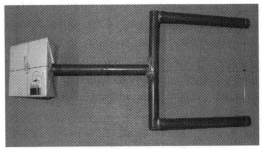

(b) Photograph of the temporal calibration phantom. The LED with connector, the lead ball, the nylon wire and the plastic bracket are clearly visible.

Fig. 5.23: US to tracking calibration phantom. (a) shows a sketch drawing and (b) shows a photograph.

The motion patterns of the LED and of the lead ball as detected by the US machine are recorded and the time offset between those measurements is determined. As an additional verification step, the latency of the optical tracking system is determined (this was already done, using a different technique, in section 3.1.1). To do this, the robot's internal system clock was calibrated to the clock of the machine running the tracking server. Calibration was performed by 10,000 ping-pong commands between the server and the robot. For each command, three time stamps were recorded for $i = 1, \ldots, 10,000$:

1. Time of sending the ping (server time), $t_{i,0}$
2. Time of responding to the ping (robot time), $t_{i,1}$
3. Time of receiving the pong (server time), $t_{i,2}$

Then the differences $\Delta_i = 0.5(t_{i,0} + t_{i,2}) - t_{i,1}$ and the offset $T_0 = 0.5(t_{1,0} + t_{1,2})$ were computed. Since these differences tend to slowly drift over time (approximately one second in ten hours) and the required accuracy is around one millisecond, a polynomial of degree two is fit to the data points $[0.5(t_{i,0} + t_{i,2}) - T_0, \Delta_i - T_0]$. This polynomial, including the offset T_0, is then used to compute server time stamps from robot time stamps. Typical values determined are $T_0 = 1277830787.08483$, $a_0 = 1949.125$, $a_1 = -1.337598 \cdot 10^{-4}$, and $a_2 = 2.248379 \cdot 10^{-7}$. This results in an accuracy of one millisecond or better for about five minutes after the calibration. Using this setup, the measurement was performed and the following values were determined:

	US to optical	optical to robot	US to robot
latency [ms]	33 ± 5	4 ± 1	36 ± 6

The findings for the latency of the optical tracking system (operating at 4.1 kHz) are well in line with a latency of 5 ms as determined in section 3.1.1. We did observe, however, that the latency of the US station heavily depended on the selected parameters. To minimise latency, the following settings were used:

volume optimisation **off**
number of cycles   **minimal**
diff   **1**
DDP   **minimal**
power   **minimal**
shading   **minimal**
flatness   **maximal**

Additionally, the station's high resolution zoom mode was activated. All other parameters remained at their default values. Figure 5.24 shows photographs of the complete setup and the recorded motion traces. Figure 5.25 shows rendered volumes of the US data, both in beamspace and worldspace. The lead ball and artefacts from glue on the nylon wire are clearly visible.

Concluding, we can say that the latency from US acquisition can safely be assumed to be less than 40 ms. For the correlation experiment, the latency between optical tracking of chest markers and US tracking will be assumed to be 30 ms.

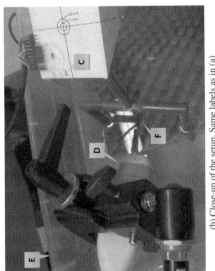

(b) Close-up of the setup. Same labels as in (a)

(c) Results of the experiment. The black curve is the LED's motion trace, the grey curve with squares is the lead ball's motion trace and the grey curve with circles is the latency-corrected motion trace of the lead ball.

(a) (A) shows the tracking camera, (B) the robot. The tracking LED is marked with (C), the US transducer with (D). (E) shows the water tank and (F) the US phantom.

Fig. 5.24: Setup of the US latency experiment

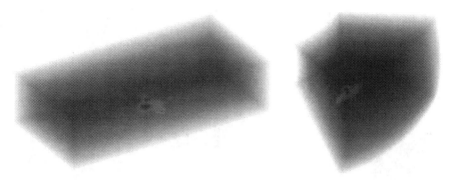

Fig. 5.25: Beamspace (left) and worldspace (right) views of the US volume showing the lead ball. Also visible are artefacts caused by glue on the nylon wire.

5.2.2.2 Data Acquisition

In addition to this setup, a volume streaming extension for the US station was written. This extension was injected into the proprietary code base of the station by patching the Direct3D Dynamically Loadable Library (DLL): whenever the station renders a newly acquired volume, the volumetric data is intercepted and transferred to the client machine via a TCP/IP connection. Using this method and a direct connection between a high-speed Linux workstation (running ubuntu 9.10 with a realtime kernel), it is possible to stream up to 60 volumes per second, depending on the volume size. For more details, see appendix C. Here, the volumetric data is sampled in beamspace, i.e., a voxel is represented by a triple (d, α, β), where d is the distance from the beam source and α and β are the angles under which the voxel is seen from the beam source. Using a nearest-neighbour lookup or trilinear interpolation, the beamspace volumes can be converted to worldspace. An example is given in figure 5.25, which shows an US view of the calibration phantom.

Using six volunteers, we acquired a total of seven data sets, ranging from 5:03 to 6:26 minutes. In all data sets, we could track vessel bifurcations in the liver. The resulting amplitudes varied from 7.3 to 37.9 mm (average, peak-to-peak). Simultaneous acquisiton of marker positions was done using a single LED attached to the volunteers' chest. This LED was recorded at a frame rate of 331.04 Hz. Taking into account the latency of the US station—as determined in section 5.2.2.1—the motion data of the LED was resampled to match the timestamps of the US data.

Figure 5.26 shows world views of three typical volumes, taken from data sets six, three, and five, respectively. Although the quality of the recorded volumes varies strongly, bifurcations can be seen in all cases. Note that the resolution of the US volumes is about 0.5 mm in all spatial axes.

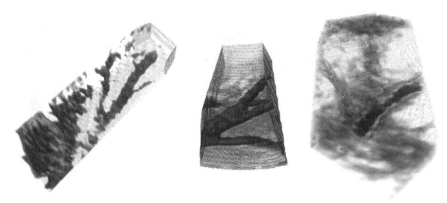

Fig. 5.26: World space views of US volumes showing parts of the liver's vessel tree in three different healthy male volunteer (data sets six, three, and five, from left to right). Differences in image quality are clearly visible.

5.2.2.3 Results

Using the data collected, we could validate the accuracy of the new correlation method. In all but one case, the new method is more accurate than the best polynomial model, outperforming it by at least 5.4 and as much as 48.7 % and by 25 % on average. In one case, it was not possible to train the SVR model such as to deliver more accurate results than the best polynomial model. The best we could get was a decrease in performance by 2.1 %. In all cases, however, the RMS of the correlation error of the SVR model was below 2 mm, in two cases even below 1 mm. The complete results are given in table 5.4.

Table 5.4: Characteristics and correlation errors (RMS) of the US test signals. On signal seven, the SVR-based correlation algorithm performed worse than the best polynomial model.

data set	dur. [min]	amp. [mm]	RMS$_{poly}$ [mm]	RMS$_{SVR}$ [mm]	gain [%]
1	6:02	11.14	1.0717	1.0143	5.36
2	5:03	14.65	1.3516	0.9237	31.67
3	6:11	29.46	1.4263	0.7319	48.68
4	5:37	37.85	3.3101	1.7690	46.56
5	6:26	29.25	2.0040	1.8609	7.14
6	6:07	7.30	1.2868	1.1511	10.55
7	6:08	18.94	1.5095	1.5407	**-2.07**
average	5:56	21.23	1.7086	1.2845	21.13

These numbers show that the SVR correlation algorithm is superior to the polynomial correlation models. Again, all algorithms were trained on a sparse set of data (three to eight points per respiratory cycle on the first 90 seconds of breathing) and remained unchanged over the duration of the signals. Although the results are very promising, we could not reach the level of improvement shown to be possible in the porcine study (see section 5.2.1). In this study, the improvement was shown to be up to 78 %. While this is unfortunate, the outcome is not entirely unexpected. Possible reasons are:

1. Inadequate resolution of the US volume. It is less than 0.5 mm, especially along the axes perpendicular to the beam direction.
2. Inaccurate tracking. We did not track possible deformation or rotation of the templates and, in certain cases, poor image quality complicated the tracking procedure (see figure 5.26).
3. Non-static US probe. Since the probe was mounted in a plastic bracket, it is possible that motion of the proband resulted in motion of the probe, therefore changing parts of the internal motion.

While the inadequate spatial resolution of the US system can currently not be changed, it is possible to take the othere problems into account and

- perform template matching with orientation tracking,
- mount the US probe more rigidly or calibrate the US volume to the tracking system to allow for compensation of probe motion,
- include deformable volume registration to detect deformation of the template.

Incorporating this into the tracking algorithm should increase both the performance of the polynomial and the SVR-based methods. Additionally, restricting possible proband motion (possibly by using a vacuum mattress) should further increase tracking accuracy.

References

[1] Ahn, S., Yi, B., Suh, Y., Kim, J., Lee, S., Shin, S., Choi, E.: A feasibility study on the prediction of tumour location in the lung from skin motion. The British Journal of Radiology 77, 588–596 (2004). DOI 10.1259/bjr/64800801
[2] Balter, J.M., Wright, J.N., Newell, L.J., Friemel, B., Dimmer, S., Cheng, Y., Wong, J., Vertatschitsch, E., Mate, T.P.: Accuracy of a wireless localization system for radiotherapy. International Journal of Radiation Oncology, Biology, Physics 61(3), 933–937 (2005). DOI 10.1016/j.ijrobp.2004.11.009
[3] Berbeco, R.I., Jiang, S.B., Sharp, G.C., Chen, G.T.Y., Mostafavi, H., Shirato, H.: Integrated radiotherapy imaging system (IRIS): design considerations of tumour tracking with linac gantry-mounted diagnostic X-ray systems with flat-panel detectors. Physics in Medicine and Biology 49(2), 243–255 (2004). DOI 10.1088/0031-9155/49/2/005
[4] Cho, B.C., Suh, Y., Dieterich, S., Keall, P.J.: A monoscopic method for real-time tumour tracking using combined occasional X-ray imaging and continuous respiratory monitoring. Physics in Medicine and Biology 53(11), 2837–2855 (2008). DOI 10.1088/0031-9155/53/11/006

[5] DeMenthon, D.F., Davis, L.S.: Model-based object pose in 25 lines of code. International Journal of Computer Vision **15**(1–2), 123–141 (1995). DOI 10.1007/bf01450852

[6] Ernst, F., Bruder, R., Schlaefer, A., Schweikard, A.: Correlation between external and internal respiratory motion: a validation study. International Journal of Computer Assisted Radiology and Surgery **6**, epub ahead of print (2011). DOI 10.1007/s11548-011-0653-6

[7] Ernst, F., Bruder, R., Schlaefer, A., Schweikard, A.: Validating an svr-based correlation algorithm on human volumetric ultrasound data. In: Proceedings of the 25th International Congress and Exhibition on Computer Assisted Radiology and Surgery (CARS'11), *International Journal of Computer Assisted Radiology and Surgery*, vol. 6, pp. S59–S60. CARS, Berlin, Germany (2011)

[8] Ernst, F., Koch, C., Schweikard, A.: A novel recording tool for education and quality assurance in digital angiography. In: 2010 Annual Meeting of the RSNA (2010)

[9] Ernst, F., Martens, V., Schlichting, S., Bešireviç, A., Kleemann, M., Koch, C., Petersen, D., Schweikard, A.: Correlating chest surface motion to motion of the liver using ε-SVR – a porcine study. In: G.Z. Yang, D.J. Hawkes, D. Rueckert, A. Noble, C. Taylor (eds.) MICCAI 2009, Part II, *Lecture Notes in Computer Science*, vol. 5762, pp. 356–364. MICCAI, Springer, London (2009). DOI 10.1007/978-3-642-04271-3_44

[10] George, R., Vedam, S.S., Chung, T.D., Ramakrishnan, V., Keall, P.J.: The application of the sinusoidal model to lung cancer patient respiratory motion. Medical Physics **32**(9), 2850–2861 (2005). DOI 10.1118/1.2001220

[11] Gierga, D.P., Brewer, J., Sharp, G.C., Betke, M., Willett, C.G., Chen, G.T.Y.: The correlation between internal and external markers for abdominal tumors: Implications for respiratory gating. International Journal of Radiation Oncology, Biology, Physics **61**(5), 1551–1558 (2005). DOI 10.1016/j.ijrobp.2004.12.013

[12] Hoisak, J.D.P., Sixel, K.E., Tirona, R., Cheung, P.C.F., Pignol, J.P.: Correlation of lung tumor motion with external surrogate indicators of respiration. International Journal of Radiation Oncology, Biology, Physics **60**(4), 1298–1306 (2004). DOI 10.1016/j.ijrobp.2004.07.681

[13] Hsu, A., Miller, N.R., Evans, P.M., Bamber, J.C., Webb, S.: Feasibility of using ultrasound for real-time tracking during radiotherapy. Medical Physics **32**(6), 1500–1512 (2005). DOI 10.1118/1.1915934

[14] Jaldén, J., Isaaksson, M.: Temporal prediction and spatial correlation of breathing motion by adaptive filtering. Tech. rep., Stanford University, Stanford, CA (2001)

[15] Kanoulas, E., Aslam, J.A., Sharp, G.C., Berbeco, R.I., Nishioka, S., Shirato, H., Jiang, S.B.: Derivation of the tumor position from external respiratory surrogates with periodical updating of the internal/external correlation. Physics in Medicine and Biology **52**(17), 5443–5456 (2007). DOI 10.1088/0031-9155/52/17/023

[16] Khamene, A., Warzelhan, J.K., Vogt, S., Elgort, D., Chefd'Hotel, C., Duerk, J.L., Lewin, J., Wacker, F.K., Sauer, F.: Characterization of internal organ motion using skin marker positions. In: C. Barillot, D.R. Haynor, P. Hellier (eds.) MICCAI 2004, Part II, *LNCS*, vol. 3217, pp. 526–533. MICCAI, Springer, St. Malo, France (2004)

[17] Kirkby, C., Stanescu, T., Rathee, S., Carlone, M., Murray, B., Fallone, B.G.: Patient dosimetry for hybrid mri-radiotherapy systems. Medical Physics **35**(3), 1019–1027 (2008). DOI 10.1118/1.2839104

[18] Knöpke, M., Ernst, F.: Flexible Markergeometrien zur Erfassung von Atmungs- und Herzbewegungen an der Körperoberfläche. In: D. Bartz, S. Bohn, J. Hoffmann (eds.) 7. Jahrestagung der Deutschen Gesellschaft für Computer- und Roboterassistierte Chirurgie, vol. 7, pp. 15–16. CURAC, Leipzig, Germany (2008)

[19] Koch, N., Liu, H.H., Starkschall, G., Jacobson, M., Forster, K.M., Liao, Z., Komaki, R., Stevens, C.W.: Evaluation of internal lung motion for respiratory-gated radiotherapy using MRI: Part I–correlating internal lung motion with skin fiducial motion. International Journal of Radiation Oncology, Biology, Physics **60**(5), 1459–1472 (2004). DOI 10.1016/j.ijrobp.2004.05.055

[20] Kupelian, P.A., Willoughby, T., Mahadevan, A., Djemil, T., Weinstein, G., Jani, S., Enke, C., Solberg, T., Flores, N., Liu, D., Beyer, D., Levine, L.: Multi-institutional clinical experience with the Calypso system in localization and continuous, real-time monitoring of the prostate gland during external radiotherapy. International Journal of Radiation Oncology, Biology, Physics **67**(4), 1088–1098 (2007). DOI 10.1016/j.ijrobp.2006.10.026

[21] Lagendijk, J.J.W., Raaymakers, B.W., Raaijmakers, A.J.E., Overweg, J., Brown, K.J., Kerkhof, E.M., van der Put, R.W., Hårdemark, B., van Vulpen, M., van der Heide, U.A.: MRI/linac integration. Radiotherapy and Oncology **86**(1), 25–29 (2008). DOI 10.1016/j.radonc.2007.10.034

[22] McClelland, J.R., Blackall, J.M., Tarte, S., Chandler, A.C., Hughes, S., Ahmad, S., Landau, D.B., Hawkes, D.J.: A continuous 4D motion model from multiple respiratory cycles for use in lung radiotherapy. Medical Physics **33**(9), 3348–3358 (2006). DOI 10.1118/1.2222079

[23] Murphy, M.J.: Tracking moving organs in real time. Seminars in Radiation Oncology **14**(1), 91–100 (2004). DOI 10.1053/j.semradonc.2003.10.005

[24] Murphy, M.J., Isaaksson, M., Jaldén, J.: Adaptive filtering to predict lung tumor breathing motion during imageguided radiation therapy. In: Proceedings of the 16th International Conference and Exhibition on Computer Assisted Radiology and Surgery (CARS'02), vol. 16, pp. 539–544. Paris, France (2002)

[25] Ozhasoglu, C., Murphy, M.J., Glosser, G., Bodduluri, M., Schweikard, A., Forster, K.M., Martin, D.P., Adler Jr., J.R.: Real-time tracking of the tumor volume in precision radiotherapy and body radiosurgery – a novel approach to compensate for respiratory motion. In: H.U. Lemke, I. Kiyonari, D. Kunio, M.W. Vannier, A.G. Farman (eds.) Computer-Assisted Radiology and Surgery (CARS 2000), pp. 691–696. Elsevier (2000)

[26] Raaijmakers, A.J.E., Raaymakers, B.W., Lagendijk, J.J.W.: Experimental verification of magnetic field dose effects for the MRI-accelerator. Physics
in Medicine and Biology 52(14), 4283–4291 (2007). DOI 10.1088/0031-
9155/52/14/017

[27] Raaymakers, B.W., Raaijmakers, A.J.E., Kotte, A.N.T.J., Jette, D., Lagendijk,
J.J.W.: Integrating an MRI scanner with a 6 MV radiotherapy accelerator: dose
deposition in a transverse magnetic field. Physics in Medicine and Biology
49(17), 4109–4118 (2004). DOI 10.1088/0031-9155/49/17/019

[28] Richter, L., Bruder, R., Schlaefer, A.: Proper force-torque sensor system for
robotized TMS: Automatic coil calibration. In: Proceedings of the 24th International Conference and Exhibition on Computer Assisted Radiology and
Surgery (CARS'10), International Journal of Computer Assisted Radiology
and Surgery, vol. 5, pp. S422–S423. CARS, Geneva, Switzerland (2010)

[29] Sawada, A., Yoda, K., Kokubo, M., Kunieda, T., Nagata, Y., Hiraoka, M.: A
technique for noninvasive respiratory gated radiation treatment system based
on a real time 3d ultrasound image correlation: A phantom study. Medical
Physics 31(2), 245–250 (2004). DOI 10.1118/1.1634482

[30] Sayeh, S., Wang, J., Main, W.T., Kilby, W., Maurer Jr., C.R.: Robotic Radiosurgery. Treating Tumors that Move with Respiration, 1st edn., chap. Respiratory
motion tracking for robotic radiosurgery, pp. 15–30. Springer, Berlin (2007).
DOI 10.1007/978-3-540-69886-9

[31] Schweikard, A., Glosser, G., Bodduluri, M., Murphy, M.J., Adler Jr.,
J.R.: Robotic Motion Compensation for Respiratory Movement during Ra-
diosurgery. Journal of Computer-Aided Surgery 5(4), 263–277 (2000).
DOI 10.3109/10929080009148894

[32] Schweikard, A., Shiomi, H., Adler Jr., J.R.: Respiration tracking in radiosurgery. Medical Physics 31(10), 2738–2741 (2004). DOI 10.1118/1.1774132

[33] Seppenwoolde, Y., Berbeco, R.I., Nishioka, S., Shirato, H., Heijmen, B.: Accuracy of tumor motion compensation algorithm from a robotic respiratory tracking system: A simulation study. Medical Physics 34(7), 2774–2784 (2007).
DOI 10.1118/1.2739811

[34] Shimizu, S., Shirato, H., Kitamura, K., Ogura, S., Akita-Dosaka, H., Tatei-
shi, U., Watanabe, Y., Fujita, K., Shimizu, T., Miyasaka, K.: Fluoroscopic
real-time tumor-tracking radiation treatment (RTRT) can reduce internal margin (IM) and set-up margin (SM) of planning target volume (PTV) for lung
tumors. In: Proceedings of the 42nd annual ASTRO meeting, International
Journal of Radiation Oncology, Biology, Physics, vol. 48, pp. 166–167 (2000).
DOI 10.1016/s0360-3016(00)80127-3

[35] Shimizu, S., Shirato, H., Kitamura, K., Shinohara, N., Harabayashi, T., Tsu-
kamoto, T., Koyanagi, T., Miyasaka, K.: Use of an implanted marker and real-
time tracking of the marker for the positioning of prostate and bladder cancers.
International Journal of Radiation Oncology, Biology, Physics 48(5), 1591–
1597 (2000). DOI 10.1016/s0360-3016(00)00809-9

[36] Shimizu, S., Shirato, H., Ogura, S., Akita-Dosaka, H., Kitamura, K., Nishioka,
T., Kagei, K., Nishimura, M., Miyasaka, K.: Detection of lung tumor move-

ment in real-time tumor-tracking radiotherapy. International Journal of Radiation Oncology, Biology, Physics **51**(2), 304–310 (2001). DOI 10.1016/s0360-3016(01)01641-8

[37] Shirato, H., Shimizu, S., Kunieda, T., Kitamura, K., van Herk, M., Kagei, K., Nishioka, T., Hashimoto, S., Fujita, K., Aoyama, H., Tsuchiya, K., Kudo, K., Miyasaka, K.: Physical aspects of a real-time tumor-tracking system for gated radiotherapy. International Journal of Radiation Oncology, Biology, Physics **48**(4), 1187 – 1195 (2000). DOI 10.1016/s0360-3016(00)00748-3

[38] Shirato, H., Shimizu, S., Shimizu, T., Nishioka, T., Miyasaka, K.: Real-time tumour-tracking radiotherapy. The Lancet **353**(9161), 1331 – 1332 (1999). DOI 10.1016/s0140-6736(99)00700-x

[39] Vedam, S.S., Kini, V.R., Keall, P.J., Ramakrishnan, V., Mostafavi, H., Mohan, R.: Quantifying the predictability of diaphragm motion during respiration with a noninvasive external marker. Medical Physics **30**(4), 505–513 (2003). DOI 10.1118/1.1558675

[40] West, J.B.: Respiratory Physiology: The Essentials, 8th edn. Lippincott Williams & Wilkins (2008)

[41] Willoughby, T.R., Kupelian, P.A., Pouliot, J., Shinohara, K., Aubin, M., III, M.R., Skrumeda, L.L., Balter, J.M., Litzenberg, D.W., Hadley, S.W., Wei, J.T., Sandler, H.M.: Target localization and real-time tracking using the Calypso 4D localization system in patients with localized prostate cancer. International Journal of Radiation Oncology, Biology, Physics **65**(2), 528–534 (2006). DOI 10.1016/j.ijrobp.2006.01.050

[42] Wu, J., Dandekar, O., Nazareth, D., Lei, P., D'Souza, W.D., Shekhar, R.: Effect of ultrasound probe on dose delivery during real-time ultrasound-guided tumor tracking. In: 28th Annual International Conference of the IEEE Engineering in Medicine and Biology Society (EMBS'06), pp. 3799–3802 (2006). DOI 10.1109/iembs.2006.260076

[43] Yan, H., Yin, F.F., Zhu, G.P., Ajlouni, M., Kim, J.H.: Adaptive prediction of internal target motion using external marker motion: a technical study. Physics in Medicine and Biology **51**(1), 31–44 (2006). DOI 10.1088/0031-9155/51/1/003

Chapter 6
Conclusion

The paramount goal of this work is the strive towards improving the technological aspects of treating tumours that move with respiration. We believe that, for optimal medical outcome, optimal technological support is required and improving the tracking and targeting accuracy of current radiotherapeutic devices is necessary.

Although many different methods for on-line tumour tracking exist (see chapter 2), focus was placed on the CyberKnife system and the CyberHeart project (see section 2.5), an extension to the CyberKnife currently under development. In this context, the current technological problems were investigated. Amongst others, these are

- system latency,
- acquisition noise,
- improving prediction algorithms, and
- improving correlation algorithms.

6.1 Analysis of Technical Problems

In the following, we will briefly outline the technical problems of live tumour tracking as listed above.

6.1.1 System Latency

From [10, 16] it is known that the systematic latency of the CyberKnife system is currently approximately 115 ms (down from 192.5 ms in an older model), i.e., from the moment the tumour starts moving until the motion has been compensated by the robotic manipulator. This latency is made up of several components:

- Phase shift (i.e., "latency") between the internal tumour motion and motion detected on the patient's chest or abdomen
- Acquisition latency of the optical tracking system used to monitor patient motion
- Processing and computing time (signal processing, robotic forward kinematics, security checks, transfer between different systems)
- Kinematic latency, i.e., delay of the robotic system

Some of these sources of latency contribute very little to the complete system latency: acquisition and computing time can both be expected to be $\ll$ 10 ms (see section 3.1.1). The main (a priori known) source of latency is kinematic latency: in our experiments, we found that even small and fast robots (like the adept Viper s850, see section 3.1.2) have considerable latencies of up to 95 ms. The last remaining source of latency, originating from phase shift between internal and external motion, can currently not be quantified: it depends very strongly on the patient and location of the tumour [14, 37, 38]. In [37] it is reported that phase difference of up to 200 ms can occur. Since this latency is highly variable and patient-dependent, it is not included in the systematic latency, i.e., it is not compensated for by the prediction algorithm. Countering this type of latency has not been discussed much, it is usually not regarded as latency but as part of the correlation model that needs to be fitted.

6.1.2 Acquisition Noise

Since it has been reported that internal motion can be much stronger than external motion [32, 33], small errors from motion tracking may be magnified significantly by prediction and correlation. We have hence investigated the accuracy of multiple tracking systems used clinically and how these errors may be reduced (see section 3.4).

6.1.3 Inadequate Prediction and Correlation Methods

The main source of error in tumour tracking and targeting comes from inaccuracies in the motion prediction and correlation algorithms. Although simulation studies [34, 40] have shown that very accurate targeting is possible using the CyberKnife and Synchrony systems, these findings do not necessarily agree with data from real patients: in [4], prediction errors of more than 1.5 mm for more than five seconds are reported; in [41], correlation errors of up to 11.5 mm in 3D were reported. These results are contradicted somewhat by [10], where mean correlation errors were stated to be less than 0.3 mm. This shows us that there must be something to motion prediction and correlation which is not fully understood yet.

6.2 Improving Motion Tracking and Tumour Targeting

As outlined above, four major fields of research have been identified: system latency, system noise, prediction and correlation methods. In this work, the last three problems were investigated.

6.2.1 System Noise

To the best of our knowledge, noise from measurement systems has not been taken into account in the current CyberKnife system. Our analysis of commercially available tracking systems show that the error when tracking moving targets cannot be ignored and that this error can become prohibitively large, depending on the tracking modality used, the distance between the tracking system and the marker, and the angle at which the marker is seen. But even under favourable conditions, reducing system noise is beneficial: it will reduce jitter of the robot motion and will improve tracking quality, since noise may be enhanced by prediction and correlation algorithms. Applying the newly developed noise reduction method resulted, depending on the algorithm, in a reduction of prediction errors by as much as 37 %.

6.2.2 Prediction Algorithms

We have investigated the performance of eight different prediction algorithms, five of which were newly inveted (the EKF frequency tracking method, the wLMS, MU-LIN, and SVRpred algorithms, and the FLA extension to the nLMS algorithm). Three other algorithms, the RLS, LMS, and nLMS algorithms were included since they have seen wide use in literature. The algorithm currently used in the CyberKnife is also LMS-based [31]. The RLS algorithm has been modified slightly such as to include an exponential smoothing term.

These new algorithms were evaluated on an extensive database of 304 motion trajectories (see section 4.5), showing that the algorithms in use clinically leave room for improvement. It could also be seen, however, that no single algorithm will be optimal in all cases: while the SVRpred algorithm did produce the best results in some cases (by as much as 50 % better than others), it also produced the worst results in other cases. On the other hand, both the wLMS and MULIN algorithms produced relatively consistent results without too much variation. The FLA extension to the nLMS algorithm showed that dynamic adaptation of parameters can be very beneficial to the prediction quality.

Comparing the three algorithms performing best, i.e., the wLMS, MULIN, and SVRpred methods, to one of the methods in use clinically, the nLMS algorithm, we can see that these three new algorithms nearly always outperform the nLMS approach.

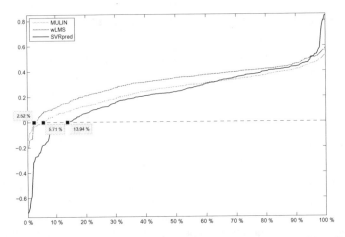

Fig. 6.1: Cumulative histogram of the change in RMS$_{rel}$ of MULIN algorithm (light grey), of the wLMS algorithm (dark grey), and of the SVRpred algorithm (black) when compared to the results of the nLMS algorithm. We can see that all three algorithms outperform the nLMS algorithm in more that 85 % of the cases, and by as much as 52 % (MULIN), 58 % (wLMS), and 84 % (SVRpred).

On average, the nLMS algorithm was outperformed by 25 % by the MULIN, by 31 % by the wLMS, and by 22 % by the SVRpred algorithm. In individual cases, the increase in accuracy was as much as 52 %, 58 %, and 84 %, respectively. The complete statistics are shown in table 6.1 and figure 6.1.

Table 6.1: Statistics of the change in relative RMS of the MULIN, wLMS, and SVRpred algorithms when compared to the nLMS algorithm

feature	MULIN	wLMS	SVRpred
maximal increase in error	14.46 %	20.02 %	71.72 %
average decrease in error	25.39 %	31.48 %	22.04 %
maximal decrease in error	52.33 %	58.33 %	83.65 %
share of signals with decrease in error	94.08 %	97.37 %	85.86 %
share of signals with at least 25 % decrease	58.22 %	73.03 %	47.37 %
share of signals with at least 50 % decrease	0.99 %	5.26 %	4.93 %

When we look closer at the best possible outcome, we see that a reduction in error by more than 50 % (i.e., RMS$_{rel} \leq 0.5$) was possible in 50 % of the cases. The complete cumulative histogram of the optimal algorithms is shown in figure 6.2.

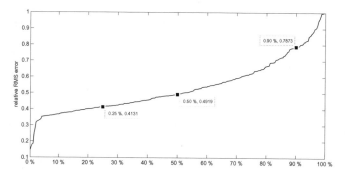

Fig. 6.2: Cumulative histogram of the relative RMS error achievable using the optimal algorithm for each signal

6.2.3 Correlation Algorithms

Since the correlation algorithm has been identified as a source of (possibly large) errors, we have investigated the algorithms currently in use in the CyberKnife and compared them to a newly devised correlation algorithm based on SVR. The algorithms were evaluated on fluoroscopic data recorded in a porcine study and on ultrasonic data recorded with the help of volunteers in our laboratory. Both experiments showed the superiority of the new SVR-based correlation algorithm in comparison to the simple polynomial models.

- In the porcine study (fluoroscopy), the SVR-based correlation model outperformed the best polynomial model by as much as 67 % when using one LED, and by up to 78 % when using eight LEDs.
- In the volunteer study (3D US), the increase in accuracy was up to 49 %, with an average of 21 %.

6.3 Tools

In the process of this work, multiple tools have been designed and developed. These tools were used extensively in our experiments but are also intended to be made available to the general public.

1. Client/server framework for communication with industrial robots and tracking systems (see appendix B and [17, 25])
2. A hardware/software solution for recording high-resolution biplanar fluoroscopic videos (see section 5.2.1.2 and [5]) as well as a fiducial tracking and calibration software
3. Client/server framework for streaming live volumetric data from our Vivid7 US station (see appendix C and [3])

4. A graphical prediction toolkit, a prediction CLI and simple batch language (see section 4.4 and [29])
5. A MATLAB GUI for feature classification of respiratory motion traces (see section 4.6)

6.4 Ideas

In the course of writing this thesis, and in many talks with other scientist at conferences and workshops, three key ideas for improving the community's understanding and progress in the field of motion prediction and correlation were identified. These are:

1. setting a standard for signal processing of motion traces
2. using a shared database of signals
3. standards for error measures and evaluation

Each of these ideas will now be briefly presented.

6.4.1 A Standard for Signal Processing of Motion Traces

Motion traces can come from a plethora of tracking devices and modalities (optical or magnetic tracking systems, X-ray-based tracking, US tracking, surface scanning, time-of-flight imaging) and feature very different acquisition frequencies (from under 10 Hz to more than 4 kHz) and resolution. This makes it inherently difficult to compare results of prediction and/or correlation algorithms based on different motion data. One part of this difficulty can be attributed to varying ideas if and how much preprocessing of the signals is allowed. In literature, downsampling, detrending, and rescaling has been used [11, 20]. We have proposed (see section 3.3) to denoise the signals prior to prediction. Since none of these methods can be employed in a real-time setting without changes to the underlying motion compensation system, these points should be discussed in the future:

- online detrending and ways of treating the trend
- resampling of the motion trace
- scaling the motion trace
- noise reduction

Ideally, a set of guidelines to signal preprocessing could be developed, resulting in a code of conduct for motion prediction studies.

6.4.2 A Database of Signals

Many works on motion prediction suffer from the same flaw: the algorithms are evaluated only on a very small sample of signals. In thirteen works [9, 11–13, 18, 20, 21, 24, 26–28, 35, 36], less than 20 motion traces are considered, seven of which even use less than ten signals. One work [22] uses 27 signals, one work uses 63 signals [39], another work 110 signals [23], and two authors use the same database of 331 motion traces [8, 30]. Most of these signals are also very short, they range from well under a minute (20 s in [9, 26, 27] and 30-50 s in [12, 13, 18, 39]), a couple of minutes (one to under four minutes [11, 12, 21, 22, 24, 28, 35] and four to five minutes [8, 23, 30, 36]), to 45 to 105 minutes [20]. In comparison, the database used in this work consists of 304 motion traces between 6.5 and 132 minutes long. More details can be seen in figure 6.3.

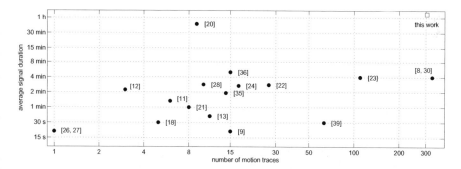

Fig. 6.3: Number of motion traces and their average duration as used in works on respiratory motion prediction. The data used in this work is marked with a rectangle.

This shows that results of different works can, if at all, be compared only with great caution. It is also of interest to look at the origin of the data: in total, there is data of eleven different origins, four from data collected using Varian's RPM system (used in eight studies), two from data collected using actual CyberKnife treatment (used in three studies and in this work), two from data collected using Mitsubishi's RTRT system (used in one study each), and three data sets of other origin (two used in one study each, one is used in three studies). More details can be found in table 6.2.

It would thus be very helpful if the largest of the motion databases (the Georgetown University Hospital signals, the Virginia Commonwealth University's 331 signals from [7]) were merged into one publicly available database. Note that the 110 signals from [23] are a subset of the 331 signals from [7] used in [8, 30].

It would also be very interesting to evaluate and compare other correlation methods (like those described in [12, 15, 21]) on the bimodal data available, i.e., the VCU_2, the OCC, and, partially, the SU data.

Table 6.2: Sources of the motion traces used. Note that most works do not use the full data sets. As an example, in [22] the first 167 seconds of the A/P motion of fourteen traces from the GUH data and seven traces from the VCU$_1$ data were used.

| | Varian RPM data | | | | CK data | | RTRT data | | Other data | | |
	VCU$_1$	VCU$_2$	RH	UMA	AR	GUH	HU	NTT	CMU	OCC	SU
number of traces	331	63	11	10	15	304	40	17	1	15	8
optical	x	x	x	x	x	x			x		
magnetic										x	
fluoroscopic		x					x	x	x		x
used in	[8, 22, 23, 30]	[18, 39]	[13]	[28]	[36]	this work, [20, 22]	[24]	[35]	[27]	[9]	[11, 12, 21]

Abbreviations: CK = CyberKnife, VCU = Virginia Commonwealth University, RH = Rigshospitalet (Copenhagen, DK), UMA = University of Michigan at Ann Arbor, AR = Accuray, GUH = Georgetown University Hospital, HU = Hokkaido University, NTT = NTT Sapporo Hospital, CMU = Carnegie Mellon University, OCC = Odette Cancer Center, SU = Stanford University

6.4.3 Standards for Error Measures and Evaluation

One standard measure, the RMS error, is used in nearly all works on respiratory motion prediction. While this measure gives a good indication of an algorithm's average prediction quality, some equally important features, like periodicity of the error, are hidden. Adopting a standard for evaluating motion prediction and correlation algorithms could also help in understanding the differences between algorithms with similar RMS errors. More specifically, the following measures would be useful:

- RMS error
- Noisiness of the output signal (introduced in section 3.2.2 as *jitter*)
- Improvement in error (called *gain* in [19] and *relative RMS* in section 3.2.1)
- Regularity of the error (introduced as *frequency content* in section 3.2.1)
- Distribution of the error

Furthermore, the question of how parameters for the prediction algorithms should be selected has not been addressed sufficiently. While it is general practice to select globally optimal parameters, i.e., those parameters resulting in the best result achievable on the complete signal, this cannot be done in clinical reality. A better approach would be

- to determine a set of globally *acceptable* parameters, i.e., parameters which should work more or less for all signals, or
- to determine *locally* optimal parameters on the first minutes of the motion trace, or

- to design automatically adapting algorithms like the FLA-approach presented in section 4.2.2.

6.5 Future Work

In the process of writing this thesis, two main fields of possible future work have been identified, namely

1. improving prediction by including additional surrogates, and
2. fusion of multiple algorithms.

We will briefly focus on these fields, outlining first ideas and, where possible, first experimental results.

6.5.1 Using Additional Surrogates[1]

During the investigation of pulsatory motion prediction, the idea of incorporating the proband's ECG signal into the prediction algorithms has surfaced. The assumption is that using this readily available electrophysiological signal would give us information about cardiac motion before it actually occurs.

Using a custom-built synchronisation board, a biosignal amplifier and a high-speed IR tracking camera, we have synchronously recorded the ECG and cardiac apex beat motion trace of a healthy male volunteer.

Pulsatory motion was recorded using the accuTrack 250 tracking system. Four LEDs were placed in the fifth intercostal space of a male test person. Using this approach, the heart's apex beat could be recorded with very high precision. Measurement noise was reduced by averaging the measured position of the four LEDs. A fifth LED was recorded to synchronise to ECG acquisition. The sampling rate was set to 1166.04 Hz, i.e., each LED was sampled at 233.21 Hz. The ECG data was acquired with a g.USBamp 24 bit biosignal amplifier [R]. The resulting sampling frequency was set to 1200 Hz, a 50 Hz notch filter was applied on the internal measurement signals in order to suppress supply frequency components. Two signals, both of approximately 30 s, were recorded using the setup shown in figure 6.4a. During recording, the proband was asked to hold his breath. Figure 6.4b shows four seconds of one of the data sets recorded.

Synchronisation of the ECG signal with the tracking data was achieved by short-circuiting the ground and reference potentials while switching the sync LED simultaneously. A fast PhotoMOSFET relay with four channels (Panasonic AQS225S) was used as switching element. The input voltages for the MOSFETs were generated by a small microcontroller board (Atmel AVR ATmega8). Test measurements

---

[1] Parts of this section have been published in [6]

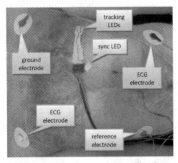
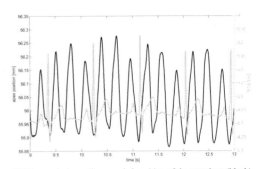

(a) Setup used for data acquisition. The photograph shows the four tracking LEDs (top), the ECG electrodes and the LED used to synchronise the ECG to the position tracking.

(b) The graph shows the recorded position of the apex beat (black) and the ECG (grey).

Fig. 6.4: Experimental setup (left) and recorded data (right)

	no prediction	w/o surrogate	with surrogate
Signal 1	0.198 mm	0.073 mm	0.062 mm
Signal 2	0.192 mm	0.069 mm	0.057 mm

Table 6.3: Prediction results of the SVRpred algorithm on the two signals recorded. The result is in mm RMS compared to the true signal.

have shown a maximum delay of 5 μs between the output channels. The delay between a state change of a tracked LED and the detection of this change by the tracking camera's software is approximately 5 ms (see section 3.1.1).

Prior to performing prediction, the recorded data was processed: both the ECG and the pulsatory motion trace were de-trended by removing a running average over two seconds. This was done to eliminate unwanted motion and DC drift in the ECG. The ECG was also smoothed using the method proposed in section 3.3.

We evaluated the performance of the SVRpred algorithm (see section 4.2.4). The algorithm was enhanced such as to include the surrogate signal for prediction. A new parameter, called *surrogate scale*, was introduced. The quality of prediction was determined by looking at the RMS error, i.e., the RMS of the difference between the predicted signal and the real signal.

Results

In the following, the numbers refer to signal one, those in parentheses to signal two.
Temporal correlation: We found the time between the occurrence of the ECG's R-peak and the next peak of the apex beat to be very stable: a mean value of 160 ± 19 (168 ± 18) ms with a standard deviation of 10 (13) ms. Additionally, we have computed the correlation coefficient r between the apex beat motion and the ECG while

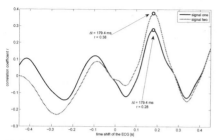
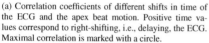
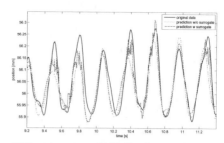

(a) Correlation coefficients of different shifts in time of the ECG and the apex beat motion. Positive time values correspond to right-shifting, i.e., delaying, the ECG. Maximal correlation is marked with a circle.

(b) Thoracic motion trace (black) and output of the prediction algorithms without (light grey) and with additional surrogate (dark grey).

Fig. 6.5: Correlation between the ECG and the motion trace (left) and results of the extended SVRpred prediction algorithm (right).

shifting the ECG in time. We found that the highest correlation can be found for shifting the ECG to the right by 179.4 ms, resulting in a correlation coefficient of r = 0.28 (0.38), see figure 6.5a.

Prediction results: We have evaluated the prediction output of the SVRpred algorithm for multiple combinations of possible parameters. Using a simple grid search, the signal history length, the error insensitivity level and the surrogate scale factor were evaluated. We found that using the surrogate will improve prediction results by approximately 15 % (18 %). The numbers are given in table 6.3 and are shown in figure 6.5b.

Further ideas

Other ideas to use additional surrogates arose from experiments performed at Stanford University Hospital, where Electromyography (EMG) data of the diaphragm was recorded, and at our department, where Electroencephalography (EEG) signals correlating to respiratory motion are currently evaluated. In both cases, initial progress has been made and promising data has been collected. More specifically, in the case of two volunteers, a correlation between low-frequency (i.e., less than 1 Hz) components of the EEG and respiratory motion was found in our laboratory. Further evaluation of this data is currently underway and new experiments are being performed.

6.5.2 Fusion of Multiple Algorithms

As seen in section 4.5, there is no single algorithm outperforming all other algorithms on all signals. It would thus be desirable to merge multiple algorithms into one to produce a hybrid algorithm possibly outperforming both ancestors. In this context, three main ideas could be investigated:

- Merging the wLMS and SVRpred algorithms into a method, where SVR is performed in the wavelet domain. This method might help in dealing with hard-to-learn signals, i.e., when pulsatory motion is visible in the thoracic motion traces.
- Using multiple algorithms in the wavelet domain prior to recombining the individual bands. Using this method, for each wavelet band, an algorithm specifically suited to this frequency range could be used. As an example, we might use a frequency tracking algorithm for the wavelet band representing cardiac motion, the MULIN algorithm for slow-changing signal parts (i.e., drift) and the SVRpred algorithm for respiratory motion bands.
- Statistical combination of multiple algorithms could also improve prediction results. In a similar way as was done with the FLA-LMS algorithms, the quality of multiple algorithms could be evaluated in real time. Once the quality of the currently used algorithm is surpassed by another algorithm, we could switch to this algorithm.

References

[1] American Association of Physicists in Medicine: Annual Meeting of the AAPM, vol. 51 (2009)

[2] Bartz, D., Bohn, S., Hoffmann, J. (eds.): Jahrestagung der Deutschen Gesellschaft für Computer- und Roboterassistierte Chirurgie, vol. 7. CURAC, Leipzig, Germany (2008)

[3] Bruder, R., Ernst, F., Schlaefer, A., Schweikard, A.: Real-time tracking of the pulmonary veins in 3D ultrasound of the beating heart. In: 51st Annual Meeting of the AAPM [1], p. 2804. DOI 10.1118/1.3182643. TH-C-304A-07

[4] Cavedon, C., Francescon, P., Cora, S., Moschini, G., Rossi, P.: Performance of a motion tracking system during cyberknife robotic radiosurgery. AIP Conference Proceedings **1099**(1), 464–467 (2009). DOI 10.1063/1.3120074

[5] Ernst, F., Koch, C., Schweikard, A.: A novel recording tool for education and quality assurance in digital angiography. In: 2010 Annual Meeting of the RSNA (2010)

[6] Ernst, F., Stender, B., Schlaefer, A., Schweikard, A.: Using ECG in motion prediction for radiosurgery of the beating heart. In: G.Z. Yang, A. Darzi (eds.) The Hamlyn Symposium on Medical Robotics, vol. 3, pp. 37–38 (2010)

[7] George, R., Vedam, S.S., Chung, T.D., Ramakrishnan, V., Keall, P.J.: The application of the sinusoidal model to lung cancer patient respiratory motion. Medical Physics **32**(9), 2850–2861 (2005). DOI 10.1118/1.2001220

[8] Goodband, J.H., Haas, O.C.L., Mills, J.A.: A comparison of neural network approaches for on-line prediction in IGRT. Medical Physics **35**(3), 1113–1122 (2008). DOI 10.1118/1.2836416

[9] Hoisak, J.D.P., Sixel, K.E., Tirona, R., Cheung, P.C.F., Pignol, J.P.: Prediction of lung tumour position based on spirometry and on abdominal displacement : Accuracy and reproducibility. Radiotherapy and Oncology **78**(3), 339–346 (2006). DOI 10.1016/j.radonc.2006.01.008

[10] Hoogeman, M., Prévost, J.B., Nuyttens, J., Pöll, J., Levendag, P., Heijmen, B.: Clinical accuracy of the respiratory tumor tracking system of the CyberKnife: Assessment by analysis of log files. International Journal of Radiation Oncology, Biology, Physics **74**(1), 297–303 (2009). DOI 10.1016/j.ijrobp.2008.12.041

[11] Isaaksson, M., Jaldén, J., Murphy, M.J.: On using an adaptive neural network to predict lung tumor motion during respiration for radiotherapy applications. Medical Physics **32**(12), 3801–3809 (2005). DOI 10.1118/1.2134958

[12] Jaldén, J., Isaaksson, M.: Temporal prediction and spatial correlation of breathing motion by adaptive filtering. Tech. rep., Stanford University, Stanford, CA (2001)

[13] Kakar, M., Nyström, H., Aarup, L.R., Nøttrup, T.J., Olsen, D.R.: Respiratory motion prediction by using the adaptive neuro fuzzy inference system (ANFIS). Physics in Medicine and Biology **50**, 4721–4728 (2005). DOI 10.1088/0031-9155/50/19/020

[14] Kanoulas, E., Aslam, J.A., Sharp, G.C., Berbeco, R.I., Nishioka, S., Shirato, H., Jiang, S.B.: Derivation of the tumor position from external respiratory surrogates with periodical updating of the internal/external correlation. Physics in Medicine and Biology **52**(17), 5443–5456 (2007). DOI 10.1088/0031-9155/52/17/023

[15] Khamene, A., Warzelhan, J.K., Vogt, S., Elgort, D., Chefd'Hotel, C., Duerk, J.L., Lewin, J., Wacker, F.K., Sauer, F.: Characterization of internal organ motion using skin marker positions. In: C. Barillot, D.R. Haynor, P. Hellier (eds.) MICCAI 2004, Part II, *LNCS*, vol. 3217, pp. 526–533. MICCAI, Springer, St. Malo, France (2004)

[16] Kilby, W.: Accuray, Inc. Private communication (Sep., 2009, and Oct., 2010)

[17] Martens, V., Ernst, F., Fränkler, T., Matthäus, L., Schlichting, S., Schweikard, A.: Ein Client-Server Framework für Trackingsysteme in medizinischen Assistenzsystemen. In: Bartz et al. [2], pp. 7–10

[18] McCall, K.C., Jeraj, R.: Dual-component model of respiratory motion based on the periodic autoregressive moving average (periodic ARMA) method. Physics in Medicine and Biology **52**(12), 3455–3466 (2007). DOI 10.1088/0031-9155/52/12/009

[19] Murphy, M.J.: Techniques of breathing prediction for real-time motion adaptation. In: RTMART Workshop 2009. Institute for Robotics, University of Lübeck, Institute for Robotics, University of Lübeck, Lübeck, Germany (2009)

[20] Murphy, M.J., Dieterich, S.: Comparative performance of linear and nonlinear neural networks to predict irregular breathing. Physics in Medicine and Biology **51**(22), 5903–5914 (2006). DOI 10.1088/0031-9155/51/22/012

[21] Murphy, M.J., Isaaksson, M., Jaldén, J.: Adaptive filtering to predict lung tumor breathing motion during imageguided radiation therapy. In: Proceedings

of the 16th International Conference and Exhibition on Computer Assisted Radiology and Surgery (CARS'02), vol. 16, pp. 539–544. Paris, France (2002)

[22] Murphy, M.J., Pokhrel, D.: Optimization of an adaptive neural network to predict breathing. Medical Physics 36(1), 40–47 (2009). DOI 10.1118/1.3026608

[23] Putra, D., Haas, O.C.L., Mills, J.A., Burnham, K.J.: A multiple model approach to respiratory motion prediction for real-time IGRT. Physics in Medicine and Biology 53(6), 1651–1663 (2008). DOI 10.1088/0031-9155/53/6/010

[24] Ren, Q., Nishioka, S., Shirato, H., Berbeco, R.I.: Adaptive prediction of respiratory motion for motion compensation radiotherapy. Physics in Medicine and Biology 52(22), 6651–6661 (2007). DOI 10.1088/0031-9155/52/22/007

[25] Richter, L., Ernst, F., Martens, V., Matthäus, L., Schweikard, A.: Client/server framework for robot control in medical assistance systems. In: Proceedings of the 24th International Congress and Exhibition on Computer Assisted Radiology and Surgery (CARS'10), *International Journal of Computer Assisted Radiology and Surgery*, vol. 5, pp. 306–307. CARS, Geneva, Switzerland (2010)

[26] Riesner, S.: Korrelations- und Prädiktionsverfahren zur Lageverfolgung in der perkutanen Radioonkologie. Ph.D. thesis, Technische Universität München (2004)

[27] Riviere, C.N., Thakral, A., Iordachita, I.I., Mitroi, G., Stoianovici, D.: Predicting respiratory motion for active canceling during percutaneous needle insertion. In: Proceedings of the 23rd Annual International Conference of the IEEE Engineering in Medicine and Biology Society, vol. 4, pp. 3477–3480 (2001)

[28] Ruan, D., Fessler, J.A., Balter, J.M.: Real-time prediction of respiratory motion based on local regression methods. Physics in Medicine and Biology 52(23), 7137–7152 (2007). DOI 10.1088/0031-9155/52/23/024

[29] Rzezovski, N., Ernst, F.: Graphical tool for the prediction of respiratory motion signals. In: Bartz et al. [2], pp. 179–180

[30] Sahih, A., Haas, O.C.L., Goodband, J.H., Putra, D., Mills, J.A., Burnham, K.J.: Respiratory motion prediction for adaptive radiotherapy. In: IAR – ACD 2006. German-French Institute for Automation and Robotics, Nancy, France (2006)

[31] Sayeh, S., Wang, J., Main, W.T., Kilby, W., Maurer Jr., C.R.: Robotic Radiosurgery. Treating Tumors that Move with Respiration, 1st edn., chap. Respiratory motion tracking for robotic radiosurgery, pp. 15–30. Springer, Berlin (2007). DOI 10.1007/978-3-540-69886-9

[32] Schweikard, A., Glosser, G., Bodduluri, M., Murphy, M.J., Adler Jr., J.R.: Robotic Motion Compensation for Respiratory Movement during Radiosurgery. Journal of Computer-Aided Surgery 5(4), 263–277 (2000). DOI 10.3109/10929080009148894

[33] Schweikard, A., Shiomi, H., Adler Jr., J.R.: Respiration tracking in radiosurgery. Medical Physics 31(10), 2738–2741 (2004). DOI 10.1118/1.1774132

[34] Seppenwoolde, Y., Berbeco, R.I., Nishioka, S., Shirato, H., Heijmen, B.: Accuracy of tumor motion compensation algorithm from a robotic respiratory tracking system: A simulation study. Medical Physics 34(7), 2774–2784 (2007). DOI 10.1118/1.2739811

[35] Sharp, G.C., Jiang, S.B., Shimizu, S., Shirato, H.: Prediction of respiratory tumour motion for real-time image-guided radiotherapy. Physics in Medicine and Biology **49**(3), 425–440 (2004). DOI 10.1088/0031-9155/49/3/006

[36] Sheng, Y., Li, S., Sayeh, S., Wang, J., Wang, H.: Fuzzy and hybrid prediction of position signal in SynchronyÂ® respiratory tracking system. In: R.J.P. de Figueiredo (ed.) SIP 2007, pp. 459–464. IASTED, Acta Press, Honolulu, USA (2007)

[37] Shirato, H., Seppenwoolde, Y., Kitamura, K., Onimura, R., Shimizu, S.: Intrafractional tumor motion: Lung and liver. Seminars in Radiation Oncology **14**(1), 10–18 (2004)

[38] Suh, Y., Dieterich, S., Cho, B.C., Keall, P.J.: An analysis of thoracic and abdominal tumour motion for stereotactic body radiotherapy patients. Physics in Medicine and Biology **53**(13), 3623–3640 (2008). DOI 10.1088/0031-9155/53/13/016

[39] Vedam, S.S., Keall, P.J., Docef, A., Todor, D.A., Kini, V.R., Mohan, R.: Predicting respiratory motion for four-dimensional radiotherapy. Medical Physics **31**(8), 2274–2283 (2004). DOI 10.1118/1.1771931

[40] Wong, K.H., Dieterich, S., Tang, J., Cleary, K.: Quantitative measurement of CyberKnife robotic arm steering. Technology in Cancer Research and Treatment **6**(6), 589–594 (2007)

[41] Wu, H., Zhang, Y., Zhao, Q., Lord, B.: Assessment of lung tumors treatment accuracy using CyberKnife Synchrony model. In: 51st Annual Meeting of the AAPM [1], p. 2463. DOI 10.1118/1.3181243. SU-FF-I-122

Appendix A
Mathematical Addenda

A.1 The à trous wavelet transform

The basic idea of this transform, called the *à trous wavelet decomposition* [6, 10–12, 17], is to iteratively convolve the input signal with an increasingly dilated wavelet function. By doing so, the original signal is transformed into a set of band-pass filtered components, so-called *scales* W_j, and the *residual* or *continuum* c_J.

We first have to choose a scaling function ϕ and an associated discrete low-pass filter h such that ϕ satisfies the dilation equation

$$\frac{1}{2}\phi\left(\frac{x}{2}\right) = \sum_{n=-\infty}^{\infty} h(n)\phi(x-n).$$

If we now assume that there is a function $f(x)$ representing the signal we want to decompose, we can define how the successively smoothed signals c_j are computed using the scaling function ϕ. Additionally, let $c_{0,k} = f(k)$.

$$c_{j,k} = \frac{1}{2^j}\left\langle f(x), \phi\left(\frac{x-k}{2^j}\right)\right\rangle, \quad j > 0 \tag{A.1}$$

The above equation can be rewritten as

$$c_{j+1,k} = \sum_{n=-\infty}^{\infty} h(n)c_{j,k+2^j n}, \quad j > 0 \tag{A.2}$$

since we work with discrete signals. Using these differently smoothed versions of the signal, we can compute the wavelet coefficients W_j by means of

$$W_{j+1,k} = c_{j,k} - c_{j+1,k}, \quad j \geq 0. \tag{A.3}$$

It is also possible to directly compute the wavelet coefficients by using the wavelet function ψ derived from the scaling function ϕ:

$$\psi(x) = 2\phi(2x) - \phi(x), \quad W_{j,k} = \frac{1}{2^j}\left\langle f(x), \psi\left(\frac{x-k}{2^j}\right)\right\rangle$$

By now deciding on a maximum level of decomposition J, say, we can deduce the reconstruction formula of the wavelet decomposition:

$$y_k = c_{0,k} = c_{J,k} + \sum_{j=1}^{J} W_{j,k} \tag{A.4}$$

Performing the à trous wavelet decomposition now boils down to selecting a suitable scaling function. The main limitation in our case is the inherent non-symmetricity of time: our time series is finite since we want to do real time processing of the measured input. This means that, if our current position in time is N, for computing the values $c_{j,N}$ and $W_{j,N}$, we cannot use values $f(k)$ with $k > N$. One thing that is commonly done to perform wavelet decomposition of finite signals is to add zeros to the end of the signal or to mirror the signal at its end. These methods, however, are not feasible for us since they add artefacts at the signal's most important part.

Consequently, the only wavelets we can actually use are those with one-sided support. The easiest such wavelet is the Haar wavelet. This is important since we want to process an incoming signal in real time.

The corresponding functions ϕ, ψ and h for the Haar wavelet are given in equation A.5 and are plotted in figure A.1.

$$\phi(x) = \begin{cases} 1 & -1 < x \leq 0 \\ 0 & \text{else} \end{cases}, \quad \psi(x) = \begin{cases} 1 & -\frac{1}{2} < x \leq 0 \\ -1 & -1 < x \leq -\frac{1}{2}, \\ 0 & \text{else} \end{cases} \quad h(x) = \begin{cases} \frac{1}{2} & -1 \leq x \leq 0 \\ 0 & \text{else} \end{cases}$$

$$\tag{A.5}$$

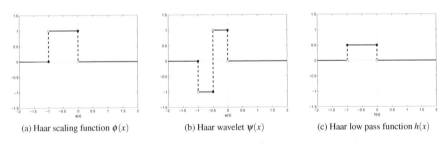

(a) Haar scaling function $\phi(x)$ (b) Haar wavelet $\psi(x)$ (c) Haar low pass function $h(x)$

Fig. A.1: Haar scaling function $\phi(x)$, wavelet $\psi(x)$ and corresponding low pass function $h(x)$

Applying these functions to equations A.1, A.2 and A.3, we arrive at the form of the à trous wavelet decomposition which we will use [7, 8]:

$$c_{0,k} = y_k, \qquad c_{j+1,k} = \frac{1}{2}\left(c_{j,k-2^j} + c_{j,k}\right)$$

$$W_{j+1,k} = c_{j,k} - c_{j+1,k} \tag{A.6}$$

$$j \geq 0$$

Example 16. Let $y(t) = 2\sin\left(\pi \cdot 0.25 \cdot t\right)^4 + 0.3\sin\left(2\pi \cdot 9 \cdot t\right) + v$ and let v be Gaussian noise with $\sigma = 0.05$ and zero mean. Let the signal be sampled at 100 Hz and let $J = 13$. This selection is somewhat arbitrary. We can now compute the à trous wavelet decomposition of this signal. Figure A.2 shows the scales W_j, $j = 1, \ldots, 13$, the continuum c_J and the relative energy content of the individual scales. This energy content is computed as

$$E(j) = \frac{\langle W_j, W_j \rangle}{\langle y - c_J, y - c_J \rangle}.$$

It is clear that the first few scales contain mostly noise, while the higher-order scales represent the actual signal. It is also clear that the higher frequency component (9 Hz) of the signal is predominantly contained in scales five to seven, while the lower frequency component (0.25 Hz) is contained in scales nine to twelve. This can also be seen when looking at the plot of the scale's energies: there are two peaks, one at $j = 6$ and one at $j = 11$. This shows that, for a synthetic signal, we can separate the signal from noise and we can also extract signal components of different frequency bands. Now it also becomes clear why J was selected as 13: the scale W_{13} is the first scale after the second peak with hardly any remaining energy.

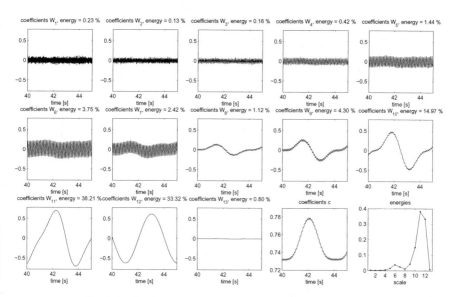

Fig. A.2: Wavelet decomposition of the signal from example 16

Thresholding and noise removal

Noise reduction of signals in the wavelet domain is generally done by modifying the individual scales W_j and c_J to form $\tilde{W}_j$ and $\tilde{c}_J$, respectively, before reconstructing the signal according to equation A.4. There are several methods to perform this modification, all based on some kind of thresholding on the individual scales. These are:

- *Hard Thresholding*: set $\tilde{W}_j$ to zero if $|W_j| < \lambda_j$ for some threshold λ_j.
- *Soft Thresholding*: let λ_j be the threshold for scale W_j. Then $\tilde{W}_j$ is computed as

$$\tilde{W}_{j,k} = \begin{cases} \operatorname{sgn}(W_{j,k})\left(|W_{j,k}| - \lambda_j\right) & \text{if } |W_{j,k}| \geq \lambda_j \\ 0 & \text{otherwise} \end{cases}.$$

- *Multiscale Entropy Filtering*: this is a method based on measuring the information content of the individual wavelet scales and subsequently trying to minimise the information in the residual $W_j - \tilde{W}_j$. More information can be found in [19].

One difficulty in the two classical thresholding methods is how the values of λ should be selected. Several ways to compute appropriate values have been presented, like the universal threshold [4], the SURE threshold [5] or the MULTI-SURE threshold [14, ch. 10].

A.2 Support Vector Regression

Support Vector Regression (SVR) is a method which, given some kind of training data

$$\{(u_1, y_1), \ldots, (u_L, y_L)\},$$

tries to find a function $f(x)$ that has at most ε deviation from the actually obtained targets y_i for all the training data, i.e.,

$$|f(u_i) - y_i| \leq \varepsilon. \tag{A.7}$$

Here, u_i is some kind of feature vector from $\mathbb{R}^M$ and $y_i \in \mathbb{R}$ is the desired output. In general, the function f we are looking for can be written as

$$f(x) = w^{\mathsf{T}} \Phi(x) + b \tag{A.8}$$

for a—possibly nonlinear—function Φ mapping $\mathbb{R}^M$ to a feature space $\mathscr{F}$, a vector $w \in \mathscr{F}$ and a scalar $b \in \mathbb{R}$. This function is now computed by solving the optimisation problem

$$
\begin{aligned}
\min_{w,b} \quad & \frac{1}{2}\|w\|^2 + C \sum_{i=1}^{L} (\xi_i + \xi_i^*) \\
\text{s.t.} \quad & y_{i+\delta} - w^{\mathsf{T}} \Phi(u_i) - b \leq \varepsilon + \xi_i \\
& w^{\mathsf{T}} \Phi(u_i) + b - y_{i+\delta} \leq \varepsilon + \xi_i^* \\
& \xi_i, \xi_i^* \geq 0, \quad i = 1, \ldots, L.
\end{aligned}
\tag{A.9}
$$

Here, ξ_i and ξ_i^* are slack variables introduced to cope with training data possibly violating the condition $|f(u_i) - y_i| \leq \varepsilon$. C controls how much these deviations are penalised. See figure A.3. Following [18], we can formulate the Lagrangian function

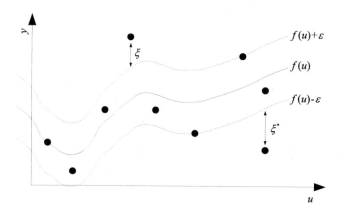

Fig. A.3: Role of the slack variables ξ and ξ^* as well as the SVR parameter ε.

of equation A.9 using Lagrange multipliers α, α^*, η and η^*:

$$\mathcal{L} = \frac{1}{2}\|w\|^2 + C\sum_{i=1}^{L}(\xi_i + \xi_i^*) - \sum_{i=1}^{L}(\eta_i\xi_i + \eta_i^*\xi_i^*)$$

$$- \sum_{i=1}^{L}\alpha_i\left(\varepsilon + \xi_i - y_{i+\delta} + w^{\mathrm{T}}\Phi(u_i) + b\right) \qquad (A.10)$$

$$- \sum_{i=1}^{L}\alpha_i^*\left(\varepsilon + \xi_i^* + y_{i+\delta} - w^{\mathrm{T}}\Phi(u_i) - b\right)$$

From the saddle point condition follows that the partial derivatives of $\mathcal{L}$ with respect to the primal variables b, w, ξ, and ξ^* have to vanish at optimality, i.e.

$$\frac{\partial\mathcal{L}}{\partial b} = \sum_{i=1}^{L}(\alpha_i^* - \alpha_i) = 0 \qquad (A.11a)$$

$$\frac{\partial\mathcal{L}}{\partial w} = w - \sum_{i=1}^{L}(\alpha_i^* - \alpha_i)\Phi(u_i) = 0 \qquad (A.11b)$$

$$\frac{\partial\mathcal{L}}{\partial\xi} = C - \alpha_i - \eta_i = 0 \qquad (A.11c)$$

$$\frac{\partial\mathcal{L}}{\partial\xi^*} = C - \alpha_i^* - \eta_i^* = 0. \qquad (A.11d)$$

By substituting equations A.11a to A.11d into equation A.10 and taking the non-negativity of the dual variables into account, we subsequently arrive at the dual optimisation problem

$$\max_{\alpha,\alpha^*} \quad -\frac{1}{2}\sum_{i,j=1}^{L}\Phi(u_i)^{\mathrm{T}}\Phi(u_j)(\alpha_i - \alpha_i^*)(\alpha_j - \alpha_j^*)$$

$$-\varepsilon\sum_{i=1}^{L}(\alpha_i + \alpha_i^*) + \sum_{i=1}^{L}y_{i+\delta}(\alpha_i - \alpha_i^*) \qquad (A.12)$$

$$\text{s.t.} \quad 0 \le \alpha_i, \alpha_i^* \le C, \quad \sum_{i=1}^{L}(\alpha_i - \alpha_i^*) = 0, \quad i = 1,\ldots,L.$$

According to [18], we introduce a kernel function $k(x,y)$ as

$$k(x,y) = \Phi(x)^{\mathrm{T}}\Phi(y). \qquad (A.13)$$

In the end, the creation of an SVR function f boils down to selecting a kernel function and solving the optimisation problem given in equation A.12. From equation A.11b and equation A.8 follows that the ε-insensitive loss function $f(x)$ can be determined as

$$f(x) = \sum_{i=1}^{L}(\alpha_i - \alpha_i^*)k(u_i,x) + b, \qquad (A.14)$$

where L is the number of samples trained, α_i and α_i^* are the Lagrangian multipliers associated with the sample pair (u_i, y_i) and k is the kernel function used.

Kernel functions

Selecting a kernel function $k(x,y)$ is subject to the condition that there is a function Φ such that

$$k(x,y) = \Phi(x)^{\mathrm{T}} \Phi(y).$$

This condition is met by functions k satisfying Mercer's Theorem [15] which states that any continuous, symmetric, positive semi-definite kernel function $k(x,y)$ can be expressed as a dot product in a high-dimensional space.
Typically, the following kernel functions are used:

- linear, i.e. $k(x,y) = \langle x,y \rangle$,
- polynomial, i.e. $k(x,y) = (\sigma \langle x,y \rangle + \tau)^n$,
- Gaussian RBF, i.e. $k(x,y) = \exp\left(-\frac{\|x-y\|_2^2}{2\sigma^2}\right)$,
- Exponential RBF, i.e. $k(x,y) = \exp\left(-\frac{\|x-y\|_1^2}{2\sigma^2}\right)$
- Hyperbolic tangent, i.e. $k(x,y) = \tanh\left(\sigma \langle x,y \rangle + \tau\right)$

Here, the values σ, τ and n are called kernel parameters. These parameters can be selected arbitrarily for all kernels but for the Multi-Layer Perceptron (MLP) kernel. Conditions for the hyperbolic tangent's parameters are given in [1].

The Accurate Online Support Vector Regression algorithm

The Accurate Online Support Vector Regression (AOSVR) library implements the algorithm for incremental and decremental support vector learning introduced in [13].
Let us come back to equation A.14 and let $\theta_i = \alpha_i - \alpha_i^*$. Note that, due to the Karush-Kuhn-Tucker (KKT) conditions (see section A.3) derived from equation A.12, at most one of α_i and α_i^* can be non-zero and both must be non-negative. Hence they both are determined uniquely by the value of θ_i. Adding a new sample (u_c, y_c) to an already trained SVR function then works as follows:

- Start off with $\theta_c = 0$. The new sample does not yet contribute to the cost function.
- Iteratively change θ_c until the new sample meets the KKT conditions corresponding to the dual SVR optimisation problem.
- While doing so, ensure that the already trained samples continue to satisfy the KKT conditions. This is achieved by changing the corresponding θ's and—if necessary—by moving samples from the support to the non-contributing set (or vice versa).

Conversely, removing an already trained sample (u_c, y_c) from the SVR function is done in a similar fashion: the corresponding coefficient θ_c is iteratively reduced to zero – it then does not contribute to the cost function f – while maintaining KKT conditions for all samples in the SVR function. Due to the complexity of the incremental and decremental algorithms, the reader is referred to the original work of Ma et al. [13] for further explanation.

A.3 The Karush-Kuhn-Tucker condition

Consider the following optimisation problem:

$$
\begin{aligned}
&\min && f(x) \\
&\text{such that } && g_i(x) \leq 0,\ i = 1,\ldots,m \\
& && h_j(x) = 0,\ j = 1,\ldots,p
\end{aligned}
\tag{A.15}
$$

Additionally, assume that f, h_i and g_j are all continuously differentiable. Then the conditions

$$
\begin{aligned}
\nabla_x L(x,\lambda,\mu) &= 0 \\
h(x) &= 0 \\
\lambda \geq 0, g(x) \leq 0, \lambda^\mathrm{T} g(x) &= 0
\end{aligned}
\tag{A.16}
$$

are called *Karush-Kuhn-Tucker* (or *KKT*) conditions of the above optimisation problem. Here,

$$
\nabla_x L(x,\lambda,\mu) = \nabla f(x) + \sum_{i=1}^{m} \lambda_i \nabla g_i(x) + \sum_{j=1}^{p} \mu_j \nabla h_j(x)
\tag{A.17}
$$

is the x-gradient of the optimisation problem's Lagrangian. Note that, in the case of unrestricted optimisation, the condition reduces to

$$
\nabla f(x) = 0,
$$

the necessary condition of optimality for unrestricted optimisation problems. Unfortunately, the KKT condition is not, by itself, a necessary condition for optimality. Additional properties of the optimisation problem must be satisfied. The reader is referred to, e.g., the work of Geiger and Kanzow [9] for more details.

A.4 Representation of Rotations

To describe the orientation and location of an arbitrary rigid object in 3D space, multiple parameters are required: first, we need information about the location and orientation of the World Coordinate System (WCS) and the local coordinate system of the object we are interested in (called Object Coordinate System (OCS)).

Euler Representation

Typically, this information is given by three rotations $\varphi = (\varphi_1, \varphi_2, \varphi_3)^T$ and three translations $t = (t_x, t_y, t_z)^T$. The three angles, called *Euler angles*, and the translation vector define how to transform the WCS to the OCS:

- rotate the WCS by φ_1 around its z-axis to get WCS$'$
- rotate WCS$'$ by φ_2 around its x-axis to get WCS$''$
- rotate WCS$''$ by φ_3 around its z-axis to get WCS$'''$
- move WCS$'''$ by t in the WCS to get the OCS

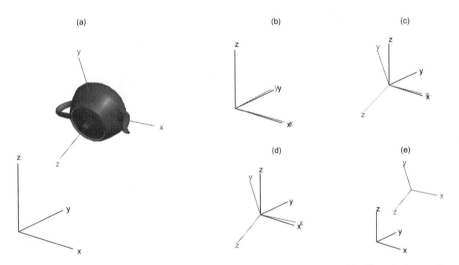

Fig. A.4: Subfig. (a) shows a teapot with its object coordinate system (black) and the world coordinate system (grey). Subfigs. (b) to (d) describe how to get from the world coordinate system to the object coordinate system: first, rotate around the z axis by the first Euler angle (subfig. (b)), then rotate around the new x axis by the second Euler angle (subfig. (c)), then rotate around the new z axis by the third Euler angle (subfig. (d)), and finally move the coordinate system to the final location by the translation vector t (subfig. (e)).

This method is visualised in figure A.4. The left panel shows the object, a red teapot, its OCS (black), and the WCS (grey). The other four panels show the four steps of transformation from the WCS to the OCS. Here, $\varphi = (3.25, 110.44, 5.40)^T$ and $t = (0.26, 1.44, 1.34)^T$.

Matrix Representation

The three rotations can be combined into a rotation matrix **M**,

$$\mathbf{M} = \text{rot}_z(\varphi_3) \cdot \text{rot}_x(\varphi_2)\text{rot}_z(\varphi_1), \tag{A.18}$$

where

$$\text{rot}_z(\alpha) = \begin{bmatrix} \cos\alpha & -\sin\alpha & 0 \\ \sin\alpha & \cos\alpha & 0 \\ 0 & 0 & 1 \end{bmatrix} \text{ and } \text{rot}_x(\alpha) = \begin{bmatrix} 1 & 0 & 0 \\ 0 & \cos\alpha & -\sin\alpha \\ 0 & \sin\alpha & \cos\alpha \end{bmatrix}. \tag{A.19}$$

This can be combined into the matrix

$$\mathbf{M} = \begin{bmatrix} c\varphi_3 \cdot c\varphi_1 - s\varphi_3 \cdot c\varphi_2 \cdot s\varphi_1 & -c\varphi_3 \cdot s\varphi_1 - s\varphi_3 \cdot c\varphi_2 \cdot c\varphi_1 & s\varphi_3 \cdot s\varphi_2 \\ s\varphi_3 \cdot c\varphi_1 + c\varphi_3 \cdot c\varphi_2 \cdot c\varphi_1 & -s\varphi_3 \cdot s\varphi_1 + c\varphi_2 \cdot c\varphi_1 & -c\varphi_3 \cdot s\varphi_2 \\ s\varphi_2 \cdot s\varphi_1 & s\varphi_2 \cdot c\varphi_1 & c\varphi_2 \end{bmatrix}, \tag{A.20}$$

where s α is a shorthand for $\sin\alpha$ and c α for $\cos\alpha$. By introducing homogeneous coordinates, i.e., adding a fourth component equal to 1 to all vectors, we can also incorporate the translation vector t into **M** as

$$\mathbf{M}_{\text{new}} = \begin{bmatrix} & & & t_x \\ & \mathbf{M} & & t_y \\ & & & t_z \\ 0 & 0 & 0 & 1 \end{bmatrix}. \tag{A.21}$$

Axis Angle Representation

A third way of describing the rotational part of **M** is by using the axis-angle description. Since the three eigenvalues of a 3×3 rotational matrix are $\lambda_1 = 1$, $\lambda_2 = \cos\theta + i\sin\theta$, $\lambda_3 = \cos\theta - i\sin\theta$, the matrix can be described by the rotation angle $\theta = \text{atan2}(\Im\lambda_2, \Re\lambda_2)$ around the eigenvector corresponding to $\lambda_1 = 1$.

Quaternion Representation

A fourth way of describing rotations uses unit quaternions. This method is closely related to the axis angle represenation, since, given the rotation angle θ and the rotation axis v, the unit quaternion **q** can be computed as

$$\mathbf{q} = \left(\cos\left(\theta/2\right), \sin\left(\theta/2\right)\hat{v}_1, \sin\left(\theta/2\right)\hat{v}_2, \sin\left(\theta/2\right)\hat{v}_3\right)^{\mathrm{T}}, \qquad (A.22)$$

where $\hat{v} = v/\|v\|$.

A.5 The QR24 and QR15 algorithms for hand-eye calibration

For many experiments in this work, accurate hand-eye calibration between a robot and a tracking system were required. While the algorithms proposed by Tsai and Lenz [20] or Daniilidis [3] provide hand-eye calibration which are optimal in one way, the results are not necessarily adequate: the algorithms always produce ortho-normal matrices. Since we may safely assume that no tracking system is calibrated perfectly, i.e., all such systems suffer from distortion, an orthonormal calibration matrix may not be optimal.

The new algorithms[1]

A naïve approach is to overcome this is to look at the general relation

$$^{R}\mathfrak{T}_{E}\,^{E}\mathfrak{T}_{M} = \,^{R}\mathfrak{T}_{T}\,^{T}\mathfrak{T}_{M}. \tag{A.23}$$

Here, the matrices $^{E}\mathfrak{T}_{M}$, the transform from the robot's effector to the marker, and $^{R}\mathfrak{T}_{T}$, the transform from the robot's base to the tracking system, are unknown. To compute these matrices, n measurements for different robot poses are taken, resulting in n equations

$$\left(^{R}\mathfrak{T}_{E}\right)_{i}\,^{E}\mathfrak{T}_{M} = \,^{R}\mathfrak{T}_{T}\left(^{T}\mathfrak{T}_{M}\right)_{i}, \quad i = 1,\ldots,n. \tag{A.24}$$

Typically, the robot's effector is moved to random points selected from a sphere with diameter r. Additionally, a random rotation of up to $\pm d$ degrees in yaw, pitch, and roll is added to the pose.

As a shorthand, let $\mathbf{R}_i = \left(^{R}\mathfrak{T}_{E}\right)_{i}$, $\mathbf{M} = \,^{E}\mathfrak{T}_{M}$, $\mathbf{T}_i = \left(^{T}\mathfrak{T}_{M}\right)_{i}$, and $\mathbf{N} = \,^{R}\mathfrak{T}_{T}$. Consequently, equation A.24 can be reduced to

$$\mathbf{R}_i\mathbf{M} - \mathbf{N}\mathbf{T}_i = 0, \quad i = 1,\ldots,n. \tag{A.25}$$

By regarding the non-trivial elements of $\mathbf{M}$ and $\mathbf{N}$ as components of a vector in $\mathbb{R}^{24}$, equation A.25 can be combined into a system of linear equations,

$$\mathbf{A}x = b, \tag{A.26}$$

where $\mathbf{A} \in \mathbb{R}^{12n \times 24}$, $b \in \mathbb{R}^{12n}$, and $x \in \mathbb{R}^{24}$. More specifically,

$$\mathbf{A} = \begin{bmatrix} \mathbf{A}_1 \\ \mathbf{A}_2 \\ \vdots \\ \mathbf{A}_n \end{bmatrix} \text{ and } b = \begin{bmatrix} b_1 \\ b_2 \\ \vdots \\ b_n \end{bmatrix}, \tag{A.27}$$

---

[1] Parts of this section have been published in [16].

where the matrices $\mathbf{A}_i \in \mathbb{R}^{12 \times 24}$ and the vectors $b_i \in \mathbb{R}^{12}$ are determined as

$$
\mathbf{A}_i = \left[\begin{array}{ccccc}
\mathscr{R}[\mathbf{R}_i](\mathbf{T}_i)_{1,1} & \mathscr{R}[\mathbf{R}_i](\mathbf{T}_i)_{2,1} & \mathscr{R}[\mathbf{R}_i](\mathbf{T}_i)_{3,1} & \mathbf{Z}_3 \\
\mathscr{R}[\mathbf{R}_i](\mathbf{T}_i)_{1,2} & \mathscr{R}[\mathbf{R}_i](\mathbf{T}_i)_{2,2} & \mathscr{R}[\mathbf{R}_i](\mathbf{T}_i)_{3,2} & \mathbf{Z}_3 \\
\mathscr{R}[\mathbf{R}_i](\mathbf{T}_i)_{1,3} & \mathscr{R}[\mathbf{R}_i](\mathbf{T}_i)_{2,3} & \mathscr{R}[\mathbf{R}_i](\mathbf{T}_i)_{3,3} & \mathbf{Z}_3 \\
\mathscr{R}[\mathbf{R}_i](\mathbf{T}_i)_{1,4} & \mathscr{R}[\mathbf{R}_i](\mathbf{T}_i)_{2,4} & \mathscr{R}[\mathbf{R}_i](\mathbf{T}_i)_{3,4} & \mathscr{R}[\mathbf{R}_i]
\end{array} \right. \left. -\mathbb{E}_{12} \right] \qquad (A.28)
$$

and

$$
b = \begin{bmatrix} 0 \\ \vdots \\ 0 \\ -\mathscr{T}[\mathbf{T}_i] \end{bmatrix}. \qquad (A.29)
$$

Here, $\mathscr{R}[\mathbf{R}_i] \in \mathbb{R}^{3 \times 3}$ is the rotational part of $\mathbf{R}_i$, $\mathscr{T}[\mathbf{T}_i] \in \mathbb{R}^3$ is the translational part of $\mathbf{T}_i$, $\mathbf{Z}_k$ is the $k \times k$ zero matrix, and $\mathbb{E}_k$ is the $k \times k$ identity matrix.

This system can then be solved (in a least squares sense) by means of QR-factorisation. The resulting vector x now contains the entries of the matrices $\mathbf{M}$ and $\mathbf{N}$. Note that this method tries to find the optimal entries for $\mathbf{M}$ and $\mathbf{N}$ in terms of the quadratic error, i.e., it minimises

$$
\sum_{i=1}^{n} \|\mathbf{R}_i \mathbf{M} - \mathbf{N} \mathbf{T}_i\|_{\mathrm{F}}, \qquad (A.30)
$$

whence the resulting matrices are not necessarily orthonormal. Here, $\|\cdot\|_{\mathrm{F}}$ is the Frobenius norm. We call this method the *QR24 algorithm for hand-eye calibration*.

Calibration using only partial tracking information

In some situations, the tracking camera might not deliver full 6-DOF poses. This will happen whenever the tracking system does not determine the pose of a rigid body but the location of one point in space (like the position of one LED or the position of maximum intensity in an US volume) or the probe does not provide full rotational information (like NDI's 5-DOF magnetic sensors, which do not provide the roll angle). In such cases, the classical calibration algorithms (like the ones presented in [20] and [3]) cannot be used. The QR24 calibration algorithm, however, can be adapted to deal with these partial measurements. A closer look at equation A.25 shows that it can be written as

$$
\mathbf{Z}_4 = \begin{bmatrix} \mathscr{R}[\mathbf{R}_i] & \mathscr{T}[\mathbf{R}_i] \\ 0 & 1 \end{bmatrix} \begin{bmatrix} \mathscr{R}[\mathbf{M}] & \mathscr{T}[\mathbf{M}] \\ 0 & 1 \end{bmatrix} - \begin{bmatrix} \mathscr{R}[\mathbf{N}] & \mathscr{T}[\mathbf{N}] \\ 0 & 1 \end{bmatrix} \begin{bmatrix} \mathscr{R}[\mathbf{T}_i] & \mathscr{T}[\mathbf{T}_i] \\ 0 & 1 \end{bmatrix} =
$$
$$
= \begin{bmatrix} \mathscr{R}[\mathbf{R}_i]\mathscr{R}[\mathbf{M}] - \mathscr{R}[\mathbf{N}]\mathscr{R}[\mathbf{T}_i] & \mathscr{R}[\mathbf{R}_i]\mathscr{T}[\mathbf{N}] + \mathscr{T}[\mathbf{R}_i] - \mathscr{R}[\mathbf{N}]\mathscr{T}[\mathbf{T}_i] - \mathscr{T}[\mathbf{N}] \\ 0 & 0 \end{bmatrix}.
$$
$$
(A.31)
$$

Using only a part of this equation,

$$\mathscr{R}[\mathbf{R}_i]\,\mathscr{T}[\mathbf{N}] + \mathscr{T}[\mathbf{R}_i] - \mathscr{R}[\mathbf{N}]\,\mathscr{T}[\mathbf{T}_i] - \mathscr{T}[\mathbf{N}] = \mathbf{Z}_{3\times1}, \qquad (A.32)$$

shows us that we can determine $\mathbf{N}$ and $\mathscr{T}_\mathbf{M}$ by only using $\mathscr{T}[\mathbf{T}_i]$ and $\mathbf{R}_i$, i.e., without rotational information from the tracking system. Consequently, the matrices $\mathbf{A}_i$ and vectors b_i from equation A.30 are changed to

$$\mathbf{A}_i = \left[\,\mathscr{R}[\mathbf{R}_i]\,(\mathbf{T}_i)_{1,4} \;\; \mathscr{R}[\mathbf{R}_i]\,(\mathbf{T}_i)_{2,4} \;\; \mathscr{R}[\mathbf{R}_i]\,(\mathbf{T}_i)_{3,4} \;\; \mathscr{R}[\mathbf{R}_i]\; -\mathbb{E}_3\,\right] \text{ and } b = -\mathscr{T}[\mathbf{R}_i].$$
$$(A.33)$$

This method is called the *QR15 algorithm for hand-eye calibration*.

Orthonormalisation

Since—as described earlier—$\mathbf{M}$ and $\mathbf{N}$ need not be orthonormal, poses calibrated using these matrices must be orthonormalised. To avoid the bias incurred by Gram-Schmidt orthonormalisation, we propose to use orthonormalisation by means of Singular Value Decomposition (SVD). To this end, let us assume that T is a pose measured by the tracking system and we want to know this pose in robot coordinates. We then compute MT, a non-orthonormal matrix, and subsequently determine the "closest" orthonormal matrix, $(MT)^{\perp}$. Let $U\Sigma V^{\mathrm{T}} = MT$ be the SVD of MT. Then $(MT)^{\perp}$ can be computed as UV^{T}.

Preconditioning the equation system

One major drawback of the QR24 algorithm is that all elements of $\mathbf{M}$ and $\mathbf{N}$ are treated equally, i.e., errors in the rotational part are treated with the same importance as errors in the translational part. But since typical tracking and rotational matrices have translations of up to 2,000 mm and the components of the rotation matrix are in $[-1, 1]$, an error of 0.1, say, is much more severe in the rotational than in the translational part.
We have thus modified the QR24 algorithm by scaling the translations by 0.001, i.e., translations are used in metres instead of millimetres. The modified algorithm will be called *QR24M*.

Computing calibration errors

Using the calibration matrices $^{\mathbf{R}}\mathfrak{T}_{\mathbf{T}}$ and $^{\mathbf{E}}\mathfrak{T}_{\mathbf{M}}$, computed by some hand-eye calibration method, we can determine the calibration quality by looking at equation A.23. In the situation of perfect calibration, this equation can be transformed to

$$\left(^{\mathbf{E}}\mathfrak{T}_{\mathbf{M}}\right)^{-1}\left(^{\mathbf{R}}\mathfrak{T}_{\mathbf{E}}\right)^{-1}\,{}^{\mathbf{R}}\mathfrak{T}_{\mathbf{T}}{}^{\mathbf{T}}\mathfrak{T}_{\mathbf{M}} \approx \mathbb{E}_4. \qquad (A.34)$$

In those cases where the tracking system does not deliver full 6-DOF results, we have to use the following equation:

$$\mathscr{T}\left[{}^{\mathbf{E}}\mathfrak{T}_{\mathbf{M}}\right] \approx \left({}^{\mathbf{R}}\mathfrak{T}_{\mathbf{E}}\right)^{-1}{}^{\mathbf{R}}\mathfrak{T}_{\mathbf{T}}\,\mathscr{T}\left[{}^{\mathbf{T}}\mathfrak{T}_{\mathbf{M}}\right] \tag{A.35}$$

Since we neither have perfect calibration nor perfect measurements, equality in the above equations does not hold. To determine calibration quality, we introduce the following measures:

- Translational accuracy
- Rotational accuracy

Let $\mathbf{A} = \left({}^{\mathbf{E}}\mathfrak{T}_{\mathbf{M}}\right)^{-1}\left({}^{\mathbf{R}}\mathfrak{T}_{\mathbf{E}}\right)^{-1}{}^{\mathbf{R}}\mathfrak{T}_{\mathbf{T}}{}^{\mathbf{T}}\mathfrak{T}_{\mathbf{M}}$. Then its translational error is defined as

$$e_{\text{trans}}[\mathbf{A}] = \sqrt{\mathbf{A}_{1,4}^2 + \mathbf{A}_{2,4}^2 + \mathbf{A}_{3,4}^2}. \tag{A.36}$$

To determine the rotational accuracy, let (θ, a) be the axis-angle representation of $\mathscr{R}[\mathbf{A}]$ (see section A.4). Then the rotation error is defined as

$$e_{\text{rot}}[\mathbf{A}] = |\theta|. \tag{A.37}$$

Clearly, this approach is only possible if both calibration matrices ${}^{\mathbf{R}}\mathfrak{T}_{\mathbf{T}}$ and ${}^{\mathbf{E}}\mathfrak{T}_{\mathbf{M}}$ as well as 6-DOF tracking information is available. If the tracking system only delivers 3-DOF or 5-DOF information, we cannot compute the rotation errors and the formula for computation of the translation error is changed to

$$e_{\text{trans}}[a] = \sqrt{a_1^2 + a_2^2 + a_3^2}, \tag{A.38}$$

where

$$a = \left({}^{\mathbf{R}}\mathfrak{T}_{\mathbf{E}}\right)^{-1}{}^{\mathbf{R}}\mathfrak{T}_{\mathbf{T}}\,\mathscr{T}\left[{}^{\mathbf{T}}\mathfrak{T}_{\mathbf{M}}\right] - \mathscr{T}\left[{}^{\mathbf{E}}\mathfrak{T}_{\mathbf{M}}\right]. \tag{A.39}$$

Comparing the algorithms

To determine the quality of the proposed calibration methods, we have performed multiple hand-eye calibration tests. In the first test, simulated data was used. In a second test, calibration was performed using a real world setup as shown in figure A.5.

Computer-generated data

To test the calibration algorithms, random matrices $\mathbf{M}$ and $\mathbf{N}$ were generated. To generate realistic values, $\mathscr{T}[\mathbf{N}]$ was selected as approximately 10 to 20 times larger than $\mathscr{T}[\mathbf{M}]$. Using these matrices, 1,000 completely random robot poses $\mathbf{R}_i$ were

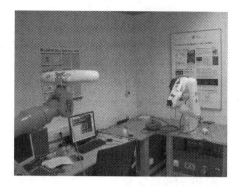 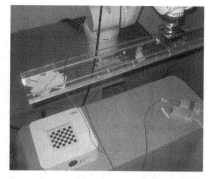

Fig. A.5: Setup of the calibration experiment (using optical tracking, left, and magnetic tracking, right). The tracking camera is mounted to a KUKA KR16 robot, the field generator is placed on a plastic table. Also shown is an adept Viper s850 robot which carries an optical four-LED marker or an acrylic bar with attached magnetic sensors.

generated and, subsequently, the corresponding tracking matrices $\mathbf{T}_i$ were computed. Both the robot and tracking matrices were corrupted using Gaussian noise in all axes of the translational part ($\sigma = 0.05mm$). The rotational part was disturbed by multiplication with a random rotation matrix around an arbitrary axis. The rotation angle was selected from a Gaussian distribution with $\sigma = 0.05°$.

Real data

Real data was generated using two tracking systems: an optical system (NDI Spectra) and a magnetic system (NDI Aurora). The Spectra was mounted to a KUKA KR 16 robot and an active four-LED marker was attached to the effector of an adept Viper s850 robot. The marker and camera were positioned such that the marker's tracked position was in the centre of the camera's working volume (in this case, at $x = 0$, $y = 0$, and $z = -1,500$ mm). Subsequently, the marker was moved to 1,000 poses around the initial pose $\mathbf{P}_0$. These poses were determined by

$$\mathbf{P}_i = \mathbf{P}_0 \mathbf{T}(t) \mathbf{R}_X(\theta_1) \mathbf{R}_Y(\theta_2) \mathbf{R}_Z(\theta_3), \quad i = 1, \dots, 1000, \qquad (A.40)$$

where $\mathbf{R}_a(\theta)$ is a rotation matrix around the a-axis by θ and $\mathbf{T}$ is a translation matrix with translation vector t. t and θ_j, $j = 1, \dots, 3$, were selected randomly for each pose $\mathbf{P}_i$ such that $\|x\| \leq r$ and $|\theta_j| \leq \theta_{max}$. r was selected as 100 mm and θ_{max} was selected as $10°$.

The values of the magnetic system were generated similarly: the field generator was placed on a plastic table and the sensor coil was attached to an acrylic plate (1 m long) which was attached to the robot's effector.

Evaluation

To compare the quality of the calibration algorithms, calibration was performed using the poses $\mathbf{P}_1, \ldots, \mathbf{P}_n$ for $n = 5, \ldots, 500$. For all such cases, the determined calibration matrices were evaluated using the remaining poses $\mathbf{P}_{501}, \ldots, \mathbf{P}_{1,000}$. The scaling, rotation and translation errors were computed for each testing pose and the average and RMS over all 500 poses was determined. Figure A.6 shows these averages for the simulated setup (top), the optical setup (centre) and the magnetic setup (bottom).

In the case of the simulated data, we could also determine the expected errors using the true matrices $\mathbf{M}$ and $\mathbf{N}$. These values are shown in light blue in figure A.6. Additionally, it was possible to determine how fast the algorithms converge to the correct matrices. The results are shown in figure A.7.

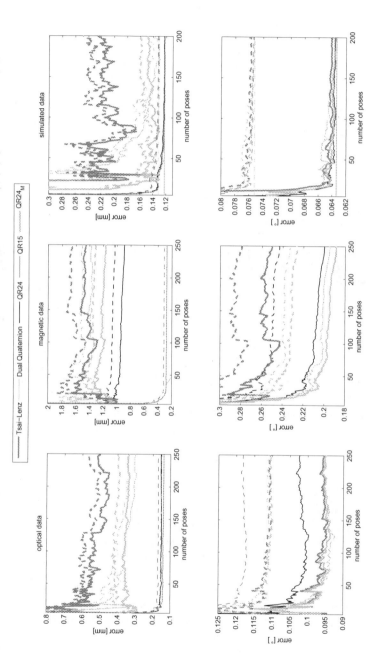

Fig. A.6: Calibration errors for the QR, Tsai-Lenz, and Dual Quaternion algorithms. The algorithms used $n = 5, \ldots, 500$ poses to compute the calibration matrices which were then tested on 500 other poses. The left graphs show the errors using optical tracking, the centre graphs show the errors using magnetic tracking, and the right graphs show the errors using simulated data. Dashed lines show the RMS of the errors on all test data, solid lines show the average of the errors. In the right graphs, the light blue lines show the calibration errors obtained using the correct matrices M and N. Only the first 250 (optical and magnetic tests) or 200 (simulation) pose pairs are shown.

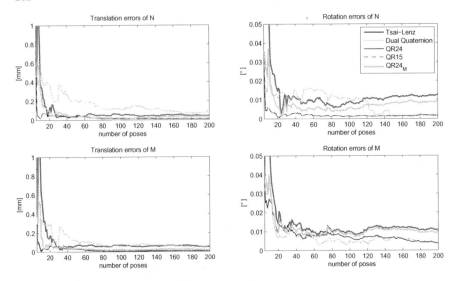

Fig. A.7: Convergence properties of the QR, Tsai-Lenz, and Dual Quaternion algorithms. The graphs show the errors between the calibration matrices M and N as computed by the respective algorithms and the true matrices.

References

[1] Burges, C.J.C.: Advances in kernel methods: support vector learning, chap. Geometry and invariance in kernel based methods, pp. 89–116. MIT Press, Cambridge, MA (1999)

[2] Combes, J.M., Grossmann, A., Tchamitchian, P. (eds.): Wavelets: Time-Frequency Methods and Phase Space. Proceedings of the International Conference. Springer, Marseille, France (1987)

[3] Daniilidis, K.: Hand-eye calibration using dual quaternions. International Journal of Robotics Research **18**(3), 286–298 (1999). DOI 10.1177/02783649922066213

[4] Donoho, D.L., Johnstone, I.M.: Ideal spatial adaptation by wavelet shrinkage. Biometrika **81**(3), 425–455 (1994). DOI 10.1093/biomet/81.3.425

[5] Donoho, D.L., Johnstone, I.M.: Adapting to unknown smoothness via wavelet shrinkage. Journal of the American Statistical Association **90**(432), 1200–1224 (1995)

[6] Dutilleux, P.: An implementation of the algorithme à trous to compute the wavelet transform. In: Combes et al. [2], pp. 298–304

[7] Ernst, F., Bruder, R., Schlaefer, A.: Processing of respiratory signals from tracking systems for motion compensated IGRT. In: 49th Annual Meeting of the AAPM, *Medical Physics*, vol. 34, p. 2565. American Association of Physicists in Medicine, Minneapolis-St. Paul, MN, USA (2007). DOI 10.1118/1.2761413. TU-EE-A3-4

[8] Ernst, F., Schlaefer, A., Schweikard, A.: Processing of respiratory motion traces for motion-compensated radiotherapy. Medical Physics 37(1), 282–294 (2010). DOI 10.1118/1.3271684

[9] Geiger, C., Kanzow, C.: Theorie und Numerik restringierter Optimierungsaufgaben. Springer Lehrbuch. Springer, Berlin, Heidelberg, New York (2002)

[10] Holschneider, M., Kronland-Martinet, R., Morlet, J., Tchamitchian, P.: A realtime algorithm for signal analysis with the help of the wavelet transform. In: Combes et al. [2], pp. 286–297

[11] Holschneider, M., Kronland-Martinet, R., Morlet, J., Tchamitchian, P.: The "algorithme ã trous". Tech. Rep. CPT-88/P.2115, Centre de Physique Théorique, CNRS Luminy (1988)

[12] Kronland-Martinet, R., Morlet, J., Grossmann, A.: Analysis of sound patterns through wavelet transforms. International Journal of Pattern Recognition and Artificial Intelligence 1(2), 273–302 (1987). DOI 10.1142/S0218001487000205

[13] Ma, J., Theiler, J., Perkins, S.: Accurate on-line support vector regression. Neural Computation 15(11), 2683–2703 (2003). DOI 10.1162/089976603322385117

[14] Mallat, S.: A wavelet tour of signal processing, 2 edn. Academic Press, San Diego (1999)

[15] Mercer, J.: Functions of positive and negative type, and their connection with the theory of integral equations. Philosophical Transactions of the Royal Society of London. Series A, Containing Papers of a Mathematical or Physical Character 209(441-458), 415–446 (1909). DOI 10.1098/rsta.1909.0016

[16] Richter, L., Ernst, F., Schlaefer, A., Schweikard, A.: Robust robot-camera calibration for robotized transcranial magnetic stimulation. The International Journal of Medical Robotics and Computer Assisted Surgery 7, epub ahead of print (2011). DOI 10.1002/rcs.411

[17] Shensa, M.J.: The discrete wavelet transform: wedding the ã trous and Mallat algorithms. IEEE Transactions on Signal Processing 40(10), 2464–2482 (1992). DOI 10.1109/78.157290

[18] Smola, A.J., Schölkopf, B.: A tutorial on support vector regression. Statistics and Computing 14, 199–222 (2004)

[19] Starck, J.L., Murtagh, F.: Multiscale entropy filtering. Signal Processing 76(2), 147–165 (1999). DOI 10.1016/s0165-1684(99)00005-5

[20] Tsai, R.Y., Lenz, R.K.: A new technique for fully autonomous and efficient 3D robotics hand/eye calibration. IEEE Transactions on Robotics and Automation 5(3), 345–358 (1989). DOI 10.1109/70.34770

Appendix B
Robots and Tracking Systems

For the experiments in this work, a variety of robots and tracking systems has been used. For simulating the CyberKnife®, a KUKA KR16 robot was used, for determining the accuracy of tracking systems and for simulating human respiratory and pulsatory motion, three different robots were used: Adept Viper s850, KUKA KR3, Kawasaki FS03N. To measure positions and orientations in space, multiple tracking devices were available. They are NDI's Aurora, Polaris, Vicra and Spectra systems, Claron Technology's MicronTracker2 H40 and S60, BIG's Flashpoint 5000, atracsys' accuTrack 250 and Ascension Technology's 3D Guidance with mid range and flat transmitters.

All tracking systems were interfaced using a common tracking framework (presented in [1]). Using this framework, it is possible to use any tracking system without any changes to the programme requiring the tracking data. The framework supports the tracking devices listed in table B.1. All servers are available as stand-alone CLI programmes and as dynamically loadable DLLs. Additionally, a graphical front-end for the server DLLs has also been designed. Using this front-end (see figure B.1), the server's output can be visualised more easily and its parameters can be set in a user-friendly way.

The robots were controlled using a common client/server architecture (rob6server, presented in [2]), which in turn connects to the robots using either RS-232 or TCP/IP connections, see table B.2.

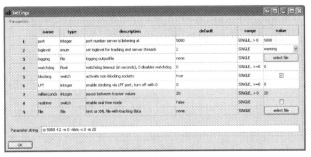

(a) Parameter setting dialog

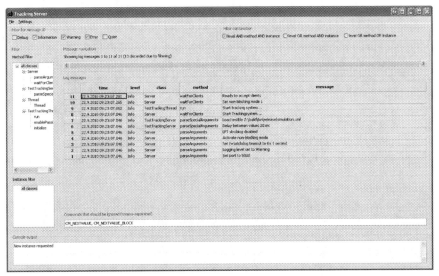

(b) Log message view with options for filtering these messages

Fig. B.1: Graphical front-end for the tracking servers

Table B.1: Tracking systems, connection modalities and operating systems supported by the tracking framework

device name	connection type	operating system				
		Windows		Linux		MacOS X
		i386	x64	i368	x64	
accuTrack	USB	✓	✓	✓	$(✓)^1$	$(✓)^1$
Vicra	USB	✓	—	$(✓)^2$	$(✓)^2$	$(✓)^2$
Spectra	USB	✓	—	$(✓)^2$	$(✓)^2$	$(✓)^2$
Polaris Classic	RS-232	✓	✓	✓	✓	✓
Aurora	RS-232	✓	✓	✓	✓	✓
MicronTracker2	FireWire	✓	—	✓	—	—
Flashpoint	RS-232	✓	✓	✓	✓	✓
3D Guidance	USB	✓	?	—	—	—
Simulator	n/a	✓	✓	✓	✓	✓

[1] The ATL library has only been experimentally compiled in our laboratory.
[2] The framework will work if the NDI host USB driver can be installed successfully.

Table B.2: Robots supported by `rob6server`, additional features and requirements

robot type	connection type	additional features	requirements
Adept Viper s850	TCP/IP	servoelectric gripper suction cup	custom programme running on the robot controller
KUKA KR3	RS-232 TCP/IP	—	proprietary driver (legacy) Ethernet RSI XML
KUKA KR16	RS-232 TCP/IP	—	proprietary driver (legacy) Ethernet RSI XML
Kawasaki FS03N	TCP/IP	—	—

accuTrack 250

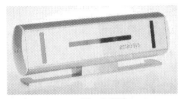

vendor	Atracsys LLC Le Mont-sur-Lausanne, Switzerland
modality	active IR, line cameras
tracking rate	up to 4,111.84 Hz single LED
interface	USB, parallel output
operating systems	Windows XP Linux (32 bit)
driver required	yes
driver open source	no

Atracsys accuTrack 250 system,
photograph courtesy of Atracsys LLC

Fig. B.2: Atracsys accuTrack 250

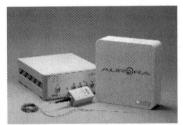

Aurora

vendor	Northern Digital, Inc. Waterloo, ON, Canada
modality	magnetic
tracking rate	40 Hz
interface	RS-232
operating systems	all
driver required	no
driver open source	—

Aurora, photograph courtesy of
Northern Digital, Inc.

Fig. B.3: NDI Aurora

Polaris Classic

vendor	Northern Digital, Inc. Waterloo, ON, Canada
modality	active and passive IR, CCDs
tracking rate	30, 45 or 60 Hz
interface	RS-232
operating systems	all
driver required	no
driver open source	—

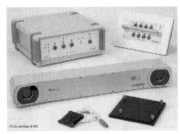

Polaris Classic, photograph courtesy of
Northern Digital, Inc.

Fig. B.4: NDI Polaris Classic

Polaris Spectra

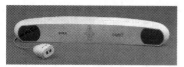

Polaris Spectra, photograph courtesy
of Northern Digital, Inc.

vendor	Northern Digital, Inc. Waterloo, ON, Canada
modality	active and passive IR, CCDs
tracking rate	30, 45 or 60 Hz
interface	USB to RS-232 host converter RS-232
operating systems (USB)	Windows XP (32 bit only) Linux with limitations
operating systems (RS232)	all
driver required	yes (USB) / no (RS-232)
driver open source	no (USB) / — (RS-232)

Fig. B.5: NDI Polaris Spectra

Polaris Vicra

vendor	Northern Digital, Inc. Waterloo, ON, Canada
modality	passive IR, CCDs
tracking rate	20 Hz
interface	USB to RS-232 host converter
operating systems	Windows XP (32 bit only) Linux with limitations
driver required	yes (USB converter)
driver open source	no

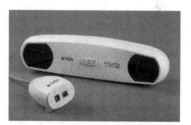

Polaris Vicra, photograph courtesy of
Northern Digital, Inc.

Fig. B.6: NDI Polaris Vicra

MicronTracker2 H40, S60

vendor	Claron Technology, Inc. Toronto, ON, Canada
modality	visible light, CCDs
tracking rate	15 Hz (H40), 30 Hz (S60)
interface	FireWire
operating systems	Windows XP (32 bit only) Linux
driver required	yes
driver open source	yes (partially)

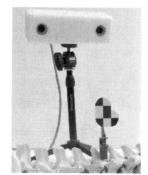

MicronTracker2 H40/S60, photograph
courtesy of Claron Technology, Inc.

Fig. B.7: Claron MicronTracker2

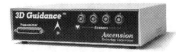

Ascension 3D Guidance (source:
www.ascension-tech.com)

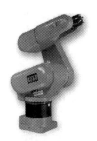

Ascension transmitters (source:
www.ascension-tech.com)

Ascension 3D Guidance

vendor	Ascension Technology Corp. Burlington, VT, USA
modality	magnetic
tracking rate	40.5 Hz (flat transmitter) 68.3 Hz (mid range transmitter)
interface	USB and RS-232
operating systems	Windows XP (USB), all (RS-232)
driver required	yes (USB) / no (RS-232)
driver open source	no / —

Fig. B.8: Ascension 3D Guidance

Flashpoint 5000

vendor	Boulder Innovation Group, Inc. Boulder, CO, USA
modality	active IR, line cameras
tracking rate	approximately 18 Hz[a]
interface	RS-232
operating systems	all
driver required	no
driver open source	—

[a] Higher tracking rates are possible, but only at the expense of risking damage to the hardware

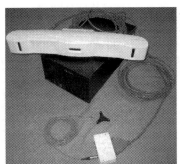

Flashpoint 5000

Fig. B.9: BIG Flashpoint 5000

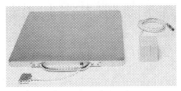

KUKA KR3
(photograph courtesy of
KUKA Roboter GmbH)

KUKA KR3

vendor	KUKA Roboter GmbH Augsburg, Germany
payload	3 kg
working envelope volume	0.679 m³, reach 635 mm
repeatability	0.05 mm

Fig. B.10: KUKA KR3

KUKA KR16

vendor	KUKA Roboter GmbH Augsburg, Germany
payload	16 kg
working envelope volume	14.5 m³, reach 1610 mm
repeatability	0.1 mm

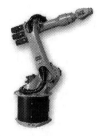

KUKA KR16
(photograph courtesy of
KUKA Roboter GmbH)

Fig. B.11: KUKA KR16

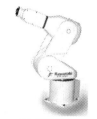

Kawasaki FS03N (source:
www.kawasakirobotics.com)

Kawasaki FS03N

vendor	KHI, Ltd. Kobe, Japan
payload	3 kg
working envelope volume	≈0.7 m³, reach 620 mm
repeatability	0.05 mm

Fig. B.12: Kawasaki FS03N

Adept Viper s850

vendor	Adept Technology, Inc. Livermore, CA, USA
payload	2.5 to 5 kg
working envelope volume	≈1.5 m³, reach 854 mm
repeatability	0.030 mm

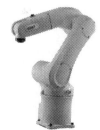

Adept Viper s850
(source: www.adept.com)

Fig. B.13: Adept Viper s850

References

[1] Martens, V., Ernst, F., Fränkler, T., Matthäus, L., Schlichting, S., Schweikard, A.: Ein Client-Server Framework für Trackingsysteme in medizinischen Assistenzsystemen. In: D. Bartz, S. Bohn, J. Hoffmann (eds.) 7. Jahrestagung der Deutschen Gesellschaft für Computer- und Roboterassistierte Chirurgie, vol. 7, pp. 7–10. CURAC, Leipzig, Germany (2008)
[2] Richter, L., Ernst, F., Martens, V., Matthäus, L., Schweikard, A.: Client/server framework for robot control in medical assistance systems. In: Proceedings of the 24th International Congress and Exhibition on Computer Assisted Radiology and Surgery (CARS'10), *International Journal of Computer Assisted Radiology and Surgery*, vol. 5, pp. 306–307. CARS, Geneva, Switzerland (2010)

Appendix C
Client/Server Framework for the Vivid7 Ultrasound Station[1]

To be able to record volumetric data recorded by our US station, a special client/-server framework was designed. Its basic implementation is outlined below.

The Ultrasound Server

Since our US station, GE's Vivid7 Dimension, runs on Windows xp, it was possible to circumvent the vendor's application and install custom programmes directly on the device.

To gain access to the volumetric data as recorded by the US probe, a specially modified version of the Direct3D DLL was injected into the system. Using this modified DLL, two system calls were intercepted:

1. All calls transferring volumetric data to the graphics card (we will call this *volume hook*)
2. All calls transferring information about the geometry of the volumes (we will call this *geometry hook*)

Once the modified DLL is loaded by the system, it starts a simple server thread providing TCP/IP access to the station at port 667. This thread also implements some basic diagnostics and the volume and geometry hook functions, which will be called whenever a new volume or new geometric information is transferred via DirectX. Figure C.2a shows a screenshot of the server running on the US machine, figure C.1 shows the server structure.

---

[1] Parts of this chapter have been published in [1, 2].

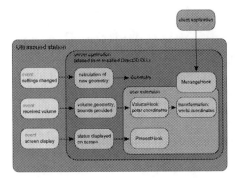

Fig. C.1: Structure of the US server

The Extensions

To be as versatile as possible, the concept of *extensions* was created. Extensions are DLLs containing code for one specific application. These DLLs can be uploaded and subsequently loaded via the server. At the moment, the following extensions are implemented:

- Debug information
- Maximum intensity tracking
- Volume streaming
- Template matching
- Transfer function upload for improved visualisation

The extension used most in this project is the volume streaming extension. Figure C.2c shows this extension running on the US machine. With this extension, it is possible to transfer data from the US machine to a client application. Data transferred includes the volumetric data recorded by the US probe, information about the volume's geometry, the ECG signal recorded, the respiratory signal recorded, and other information like system time stamps or processing time. This transfer is done via TCP/IP, using GB ethernet. Note that a typical US volume has a size of $429 \times 116 \times 16$ voxels, i.e., a size of approximately 778 kB. At a frame rate of around 20 Hz, this amounts to about 15.2 MB/sec, too much for standard 100 MBit ethernet. Additionally, the extension is also capable of computing the world volume on-the-fly, using nearest neighbour or trilinear interpolation. This conversion, however, is slow and the data transmitted will increase substantially: the world volume, sampled at 0.5 mm resolution, has a size of $260 \times 260 \times 74$ voxels, corresponding to approximately 4.77 MB. Using nearest neighbour interpolation, the highest throughput achievable then is about 11 Hz, i.e., around 52.5 MB/s. If both beam and world space data should be transferred, and trilinear interpolation should be used, the rate drops to about 4 Hz.

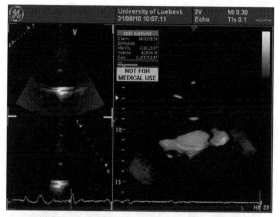

(a) Screenshot of the server running on our US machine

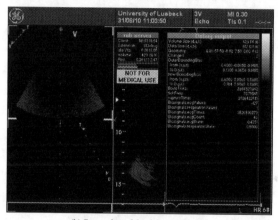

(b) Screenshot of the debug extension

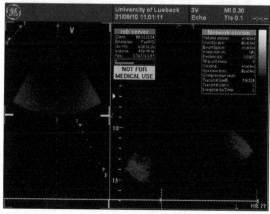

(c) Screenshot of the volume out extension

Fig. C.2: Screenshots of the US server (a), the debug (b) and volume out (c) extensions

The Volume Streaming Client

To receive the data from the US station, a volume streaming client has been developed. This client is written in C++, using the wxWidgets toolkit for its GUI [3]. The application features three windows, a streaming output windows (see figure C.3a), a station management window (see figure C.3b), and a tag list window (see figure C.3c).

In the streaming output window, the user can select where to save the data received from the US station, the output format, the number of volumes to record, and whether the streaming client should compute the world space data.

The station management window allows to manage the volume streaming extension, i.e., whether to transfer beam and/or world space data, how the world space data should be computed, and if the data should be clipped.

Finally, the tag list window shows all information transferred from the US station in the tag format, i.e., with name, data type, number of elements, values, and transfer flags. The tag list window is also used to select the tags the user whishes to save in addition to the volumetric data.

MATLAB Scripts

To be able to work with the data recorded by the volume streaming client, several scripts for MATLAB have been written: a three-plane viewing application, a template matching routine, and a fast beam-to-world conversion programme.

Three-Plane Viewer

The three-plane viewer is used to visualise volumetric time series and allows the user to select a template which should be used for target tracking in the US volumes. Figure C.4 shows a screenshot of the viewer.

Template Matching

Using a template selected in the three-plane viewer, it is possible to track this template in the 4D volume data sets (i.e., 3D plus time). This tracking is done using two steps: first, the template is roughly located using phase-based crosscorrelation or Sum of Squared Distances (SSD). Second, the location is refined by spatial crosscorrelation or SSD using interpolation and constrained minimisation. In all but the first volumes, the initial phase-based search is only done on a subvolume centred around the last detected template position. In those cases, where the crosscorrelation coefficient is too small (i.e., ≤ 0.5) or the square root of the mean of the SSD

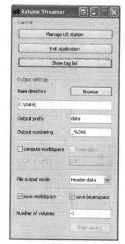

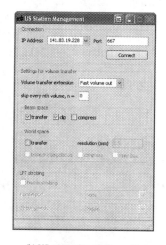

(a) Main window, with output management settings

(b) US connection window, with transfer settings

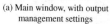

Current tags

	type	count	value	flags	save
AllTick	UINT32	1	5755		✓
BaseTick	UINT64	1	7279490338		
BeamSp	BOOL	1	true		
BeamVol	UCHAR	796224	n/a	MULTI | NMEM	
CleanTick	UINT32	1	6		✓
CompTick	UINT32	1	2389		✓
ECG	INT16	14	n/a	MULTI | MEM	
ProcTick	UINT64	1	22490225714		✓
Resp	INT16	14	n/a	MULTI | MEM	
RespStat	FLOAT	1	0.499771		
SendTick	UINT32	1	2549		✓
SrvTime	DOUBLE	1	1283248074.359218		✓
TickDiff	UINT32	1	3173		✓
Tickfreq	UINT64	1	3579545		
Time	UINT32	1	6282079		
WorldSp	BOOL	1	false		
aDatSize	UINT32	1	128		✓
aDist	FLOAT	1	0.008693		✓
aOffset	FLOAT	1	-57.497372		✓
aVolSize	UINT32	1	116		✓
bDatSize	UINT32	1	16		✓
bDist	FLOAT	1	-0.018979		✓
bOffset	FLOAT	1	7.499787		✓
bVolSize	UINT32	1	16		✓
dDatSize	UINT32	1	512		✓
dEnd	FLOAT	1	0.130000		✓
dStart	FLOAT	1	0.000000		✓
dVolSize	UINT32	1	429		✓
ecgState	FLOAT	1	0.282258		✓
ecgTimes	INT64	14	n/a	MULTI | MEM	
missed	INT64	0	n/a	MULTI | MEM	

Previously seen tags

	type	count	value	flags	save
Res	UNKNOWN	n/a	unknown	n/a	✓
xOffset	UNKNOWN	n/a	unknown	n/a	✓
xSize	UNKNOWN	n/a	unknown	n/a	✓
xWmax	UNKNOWN	n/a	unknown	n/a	✓
xWmin	UNKNOWN	n/a	unknown	n/a	✓
yOffset	UNKNOWN	n/a	unknown	n/a	✓
ySize	UNKNOWN	n/a	unknown	n/a	✓
yWmax	UNKNOWN	n/a	unknown	n/a	✓
yWmin	UNKNOWN	n/a	unknown	n/a	✓
zOffset	UNKNOWN	n/a	unknown	n/a	✓
zSize	UNKNOWN	n/a	unknown	n/a	✓
zWmax	UNKNOWN	n/a	unknown	n/a	✓
zWmin	UNKNOWN	n/a	unknown	n/a	✓

(c) List of the tags transferred from the US station

Fig. C.3: Volume streaming client

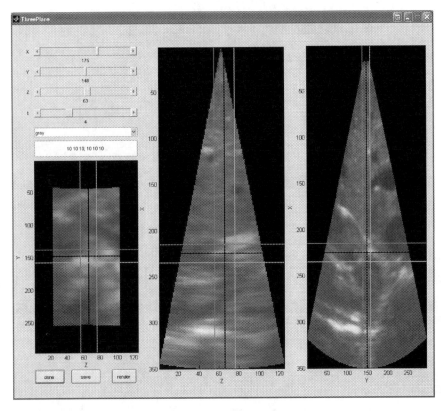

Fig. C.4: Three-plane viewer showing a 3D US scan of the liver and right kidney. The center lines indicate the currently shown planes, the other lines the template selected. Resolution is 0.4 mm, volume size is $350 \times 296 \times 125$ **voxels.**

value is too large (i.e., ≥ 50), the search is repeated on the whole volume. The US trajectories in section 4.7.1 and section 5.2.2.2 were acquired using this method.

Beam-to-World Conversion

Since, as mentioned before, on-the-fly conversion from beam to world space is too slow, we have implemented a fast conversion method using lookup tables for both nearest neighbour and trilinear interpolation. Additionally, the execution time was significantly reduced by parallelising the code using OpenMP. The conversion routine has been written in C++ and can be compiled as a .mex-file for MATLAB on Windows and Linux platforms.

References

[1] Bruder, R., Ernst, F., Schlaefer, A., Schweikard, A.: A framework for real-time target tracking in radiosurgery using three-dimensional ultrasound. In: Proceedings of the 25th International Congress and Exhibition on Computer Assisted Radiology and Surgery (CARS'11), *International Journal of Computer Assisted Radiology and Surgery*, vol. 6, pp. S306–S307. CARS, Berlin, Germany (2011)

[2] Bruder, R., Jauer, P., Ernst, F., Richter, L., Schweikard, A.: Real-time 4D ultrasound visualization with the Voreen framework. In: ACM SIGGRAPH 2011 Posters, SIGGRAPH '11. ACM, New York, NY, USA (2011)

[3] wxWidgets – a cross-platform GUI library. Available online. URL http://www.wxwidgets.org

Appendix D
Simulating Respiration

Since real respiratory motion traces are not readily available in all lengths and with all properties desired, it is sometimes very useful to simulate human respiratory motion.

The basic idea is to generate a periodic signal. This signal can then be further modified to account for the variations observed in real respiration. It is known that typical human respiratory motion has a frequency of somewhere between 0.1 and 0.5 Hz, that it has a pause at expiration and that inspiration flanks are usually steeper than expiration flanks. With this in mind, it is reasonable to define a typical human respiratory cycle to consist of two parts: inspiration is modelled as $|\sin^{e_1}|$ and expiration is modelled as $|\sin^{e_2}|$. The basic formula would thus be

$$x(t) = \begin{cases} A\left|\sin^{e_1}\left(2\pi\frac{f}{2} \cdot t\right)\right| & \text{for } t \in \Omega\left(f\right) \\ A\left|\sin^{e_2}\left(2\pi\frac{f}{2} \cdot t\right)\right| & \text{else} \end{cases}, \tag{D.1}$$

where

$$\Omega\left(f\right) = \left\{x \in \mathbb{R} : \text{round}\left(2x \cdot f - \frac{1}{2}\right) \equiv 0 \bmod 2\right\}. \tag{D.2}$$

Clearly, this is only a start: in reality, the amplitude of each cycle may change as may the position of maximum exhalation. Additionally, the respiratory frequency f will fluctuate slightly over time. To also allow for measurement errors and patient motion other than respiration, we have to add noise and simulate gradual baseline drift.

In the following, let us assume we wish to generate a signal with M complete cycles having a total of N samples such that M divides N.

Varying amplitude and baseline

Varying the signal's amplitude can be achieved by replacing A in equation D.1 by A_i for each individual respiratory cycle i. A_i can be derived from A as

$$A_i = A + \delta_A \cdot A \cdot v, \quad i = 1, \ldots, M \tag{D.3}$$

where v is drawn from a continuous uniform distribution on $[-1, 1]$ and δ_A is a parameter describing the maximal allowed change in amplitude. Baseline changes are modelled in two components: first, random changes of the level of maximum exhale are modelled as a cubic spline defined by the nodes

$$(t_i, b_i) = \left(\frac{i-1}{f}, \delta_b \cdot A \cdot v \right), \quad i = 1, \ldots, M \tag{D.4}$$

where δ_b describes the maximal allowed baseline shift per breathing cycle. Additionaly, long term drift in the baseline is modelled as a cubic spline through the nodes

$$(t_i, B_i) = \left(\min \left(t_N, \frac{N_B(i-1)}{f} \right), \delta_B \cdot A \cdot \sum_{k=1}^{i} v \right), \quad i = 1, \ldots, \left\lceil \frac{M}{N_B} \right\rceil \tag{D.5}$$

where N_B indicates the speed of baseline change (one node for the cubic spline is generated once every N_B breathing cycles) and δ_B describes the maximum drift in baseline per node. Additionally, the noise in this case is modelled additively, i.e., it is somewhat like Brownian motion with the difference that v is not drawn from a normal but a uniform distribution.

Frequency variation

Changes in the frequency of respiration are modelled by inhomogeneous resampling of the breathing cycles. For each cycle, we compute

$$T_{i,\uparrow} = 1 + \delta_T \cdot v \quad \text{and} \quad T_{i,\downarrow} = 1 + \delta_T \cdot v, \quad i = 1, \ldots, M \tag{D.6}$$

to allow for independent resampling of inspiration ($\uparrow$) and expiration ($\downarrow$). Then the time stamps for cycle i, $C_i = \left[t_{(i-1)\bar{N}}, t_{(i-1)\bar{N}+1}, \ldots, t_{i\bar{N}} \right]$, where $\bar{N} = N/M$ is the number of samples per cycle, are changed to

$$\tilde{C}_i = \left[t_{(i-1)\bar{N}}, t_{(i-1)\bar{N}} + \Delta_{i,\uparrow}, \ldots, t_{(i-1)\bar{N}+\left\lfloor \frac{\bar{N}}{2} \right\rfloor}, t_{(i-1)\bar{N}+\left\lfloor \frac{\bar{N}}{2} \right\rfloor} + \Delta_{i,\downarrow}, \ldots, t_{i\bar{N}} \right], \tag{D.7}$$

where

$$\Delta_{i,\uparrow} = \frac{t_{(i-1)\bar{N}+\left\lfloor\frac{\bar{N}}{2}\right\rfloor} - t_{(i-1)\bar{N}}}{\left\lfloor\frac{T_i\bar{N}}{2}\right\rfloor} \quad \text{and} \quad \Delta_{i,\downarrow} = \frac{t_{i\bar{N}} - t_{(i-1)\bar{N}+\left\lfloor\frac{\bar{N}}{2}\right\rfloor}}{\left\lceil\frac{T_i\bar{N}}{2}\right\rceil}. \tag{D.8}$$

Next, the new time vector $\tilde{t} = \left[\tilde{C}_1, \tilde{C}_2, \dots\right]$ is resampled to have the same number of samples as the old time vector $t = [C_1, C_2, \dots]$. Finally, the time series (t, x) is interpolated on $\tilde{t}$ to find $\tilde{x}$. Then $\tilde{t}$ is replaced by t and $(t, \tilde{x})$ is the new time series with cycles of different frequencies.

Noise

The final signal is then formed by replacing $\tilde{x}$ by $\tilde{x} + \xi$, where $\xi \sim \mathcal{N}\left(0, (\sigma A)^2\right)$ for some σ.

Example 17. As an example, the signal shown in figure D.1 was generated using this method with $A = 2$, $f = 0.25$, $e_1 = 8$, $e_2 = 4$ and $t = (0, 0.01, \dots, 100)^{\mathrm{T}}$, i.e., $M = 25$ and $N = 10,000$. The modification parameters were $\delta_A = 0.2$, $\delta_b = 0.1$, $\delta_B = 0.3$, $N_B = 10$, $\delta_T = 0.1$, $\sigma = 0.015$.

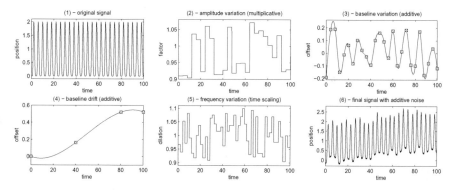

Fig. D.1: Simulated respiratory motion trace. The subplots show how the final signal (6) is built from the original signal (1) using multiplicative amplitude variation (2), baseline variation (3) and drift (4), frequency changes (5) and additive noise (6). The grey boxes in (3) and (4) show the nodes of the splines generated.

Appendix E
Listings

Listing E.1 Initial version of the SVRpred prediction method

```
FOR n = δ ;  n < NumberOfSamples ;  n++
    ' build  signal  history
    ' mode  can  be  LINEAR  or  QUADRATIC
    uₙ = HISTORY( n , M , mode , stepping )

    ' train
    TRAIN( uₙ₋δ , yₙ )

    ' predict
    ŷₙ₊δ = PREDICT( uₙ )

    ' forget
    IF  n > MinimalNumberOfTrainedSamples
        FORGET( sample ( 0 ))
    END
END
```

Listing E.2 Training and forgetting only a subset of samples

```
τ = 0.1  ' training percentage

FOR n = δ;  n < NumberOfSamples;  n++

   . . .

   ' training
   IF n ≡ 0 mod INT(1/τ)
     TRAIN(u_{n-δ}, y_n)
   END

   ' forgetting
   IF n > MinimalNumberOfTrainedSamples
     IF n ≡ 0 mod INT(1/τ)
       FORGET(sample(0))
     END
   END

   . . .

END
```

Listing E.3 Algorithm for thresholded extremal search

```
' x = (x_1,...,x_N)^T is the input data
' τ is a threshold, usually set to 0.05(max(x) - min(x))

' initialisation
currentMin = (x_1, 1)
currentMax = (x_1, 1)

IF x_1 > x_2
    ρ = 1
ELSE
    ρ = 0
END

FOR n = 1;  n < N;  n++
    IF x_n < currentMax_1 - τ ∧ ρ = 1
        M := [M; currentMax]
        ρ := 0
        currentMin := (x_n, n);
    ELSE IF x_n > currentMin_1 + τ ∧ ρ = 0
        m := [m; currentMin]
        ρ := 1
        currentMax := [x_n, n]
    END
END
```

Listing E.4 Example listing of a script for evaluation using the PredictorCLI application (see section 4.4).

```
 1   # set output level
 2   log 3
 3   # load configuration file
 4   load /home/ernst/data/20100104_herz_us/pred_hires_linux.xml
 5   # set data file
 6   eg data_filename /home/ernst/data/20100104_herz_us/volumes1939499POS_hires_mod.txt
 7   # enter custom mode
 8   ec
 9   # initialize data
10   initialize
11   # Evaluate the MULIN algorithm
12   # create 20 instances of algorithm #2 for parallel evaluation
13   rs 2 20
14   # set parameter level of algorithm #2 to 0
15   c 2 level 0 0 0
16   # timing
17   tic
18   # start evaluation
19   ev 2 /home/ernst/data/20100104_herz_us/pred_hires_mulin_0.m -1 learning 0 1 2000
20   # leave custom mode
21   q
```

List of Figures

List of Tables

List of Companies

(A) Accuray, Inc., 1310 Chesapeake Terrace, Sunnyvale, CA 94089, USA

(B) KUKA Roboter GmbH, Zugspitzstraße 140, 86165 Augsburg, Germany

(C) Stryker, Inc., 2825 Airview Boulevard, Kalamazoo, MI 49002, USA

(D) MHI, Inc., 16-5, Kounan 2-chome, Minato, Tokyo 108-8125, Japan

(E) BrainLAB AG, Kapellenstr. 12, 85622 Feldkirchen, Germany

(F) Elekta AB, Kungstensgatan 18, SE-103 93 Stockholm, Sweden

(G) Varian Medical Systems, Inc., 3100 Hansen Way, Palo Alto, CA 94304, USA

(H) TomoTherapy Incorporated, 1240 Deming Way, Madison, WI 53717, USA

(I) Best nomos, One Best Drive, Pittsburgh, PA 15202, USA

(J) CyberHeart, Inc., 570 Del Rey Ave, Sunnyvale, CA 94085, USA

(K) Atracsys LLC, Ch. de Maillefer 47, 1052 Le Mont-sur-Lausanne, Switzerland

(L) Adept Technology, Inc., 5960 Inglewood Dr., Pleasanton, CA 94588, USA

(M) St Jude Medical, Inc., 1 St. Jude Medical Drive, St. Paul, MN 55117, USA

(N) GE Healthcare Inc., Amersham Place, Little Chalfont, Bucks HP7 9NA, UK

(O) Philips Deutschland GmbH, Lübeckertordamm 5, 20099 Hamburg, Germany

(P) Matrox Electronic Systems Ltd., 1055 St-Regis Blvd., Dorval, Quebec, Canada

(Q) ATI Industrial Automation, Inc., 1031 Goodworth Dr., Apex, NC 27539, USA

(R) g.tec Guger Technologies, Herbersteinstraße 60, 8020 Graz, Austria

Glossary

3D Conformal Radiation Therapy (3DCRT)
   A treatment method in radiation therapy.

Accurate Online Support Vector Regression (AOSVR)
   A concept of online modification of Support Vector Regression Machines.
Autoregressive Moving Average (ARMA)
   A linear model for a stationary, time-discrete stochastic process.

Beam's Eye View (BEV)
   An image taken during radiation therapy with an imager directly in line with
   the treatment beam.
BMBF
   Bundesministerium für Bildung und Forschung, German Federal Ministry of
   Education and Research.

CLI
   Command-Line Interpreter.
Clinical Target Volume (CTV)
   The tumour volume which is supposed to be targeted during irradiation.
Computed Tomography (CT)
   A method to compute a 3D volume from multiple X-ray images.
Conformal Radiation Therapy (CRT)
   A treatment method in radiation therapy.
Cumulative Distribution Function (CDF)
   A function describing the likelihood for a random variable to occur at a given
   point or less.

DC
   Direct Current, i.e., unidirectional flow of electric energy.
Deep Inspiration Breath Hold (DIBH)
   A gating method where dose is delivered when the patient achieves maximum
   inspiration.

Degrees of Freedom (DOF)
  Number of joints of a robotic manipulator.
DFG
  Deutsche Forschungsgemeinschaft, German Research Foundation.
Discrete Fourier Transform (DFT)
  A way to compute the frequencies and corresponding energies present in a discretely sampled signal.
dual polynomial
  A function which polynomially models hysteresis.
Dynamic Multi-Leaf Collimator (DMLC)
  A Multi-Leaf Collimator where the leaves can be moved during treatment to account for patient motion.
Dynamically Loadable Library (DLL)
  A file containing executable programme code which can be loaded at runtime.

Electrocardiogram (ECG)
  Recording of the electrical activity of the heart as measured on the body surface.
Electroencephalography (EEG)
  The method of recording electrical activity of the brain by placing highly sensitive electrodes on the scalp.
Electromyography (EMG)
  A technique for evaluating and recording the electrical activity produced by skeletal muscles.
EM
  Electromagnetic.
Extended Kalman Filter (EKF)
  The Extended Kalman Filter is an extension of the Kalman Filter to situations where the observation function and/or the state transition function are not linear.
Extensible Markup Language (XML)
  XML is a markup language used to transform hierarchically organised data into machine-readable form. It was standardised by the W3C in 1998.

Fast Fourier Transform (FFT)
  The Fast Fourier Transform is an effective algorithm to compute the values of a Discrete Fourier Transform.
Fast Lane Approach (FLA)
  A method to automatically adapt the LMS and nLMS algorithms' parameters μ and M.
fiducial
  Artificial landmark implanted.
frequency leakage
  The effect of motion in one spatial axis being registerd in the other axes due to measuring errors stemming from active IR tracking devices.
FUSION
  Future Environment for Gentle Liver Surgery Using Image-Guided Planning and Intra-Operative Navigation.

gating
    Synchronising the radiotherapeutic treatment beam to certain respiratory phases.
Gross Tumour Volume (GTV)
    The actual volume of the cancerous region as determined by the clinician.
GUI
    Graphical User Interface.

Infrared (IR)
    Electromagnetic radiation with a wavelength $\lambda \in [0.7, 300]$ μm.
Intensity Modulated Radiation Therapy (IMRT)
    A treatment method in radiation therapy.
International Classification of Diseases, version 10 (ICD-10)
    The ICD, endorsed by the WHO in 1990, is used to classify diseases and other
    health problems recorded on many types of health and vital records including
    death certificates and health records.

JPEG
    JPEG is a commonly used method of lossy compression for photographic
    images named after the Joint Photographic Experts Group.

Kalman Filter (KF)
    The Kalman Filter is a set of equations used to derive information about a sys-
    tem's state using some kind of, possibly corrupted, time-varying observations
    of the system's output. Both the function to compute the output from the states
    as well as the state at the next time instance must be linear.
Karush-Kuhn-Tucker (KKT) condition
    A necessary condition for the solution of constrained optimisation problems.
    For more details, see section A.3.
kilovoltage (kV)
    1,000 volts.

Least Mean Squares (LMS)
    A time-recursive approximation algorithm based on the gradient descent me-
    thod.
Light Emitting Diode (LED)
    A semiconductor light source.
Linear Accelerator (LINAC)
    A device emitting γ-radiation generated by means of deflecting accelerated elec-
    trons.

Magnetic Resonance Imaging (MRI)
    A volumetric imaging method based on the principle of nuclear magnetic reso-
    nance.
Manual Control Pendant (MCP)
    A device to manually control a robot's motion.

megavoltage (MV)
>   1,000,000 volts.

MJPEG
>   Motion JPEG (M-JPEG) is an informal name for a class of video formats where each video frame or interlaced field of a digital video sequence is separately compressed as a JPEG image.

model-based prediction method
>   Prediction algorithm making use of background knowledge about the signal to predict, i.e., periodicity, speed, stationarity, maximal dynamics etc..

model-free prediction method
>   Prediction algorithm without any assumptions about the signal to predict.

Motion-Adaptive Delivery (MAD)
>   A way of delivering a TomoTherapy treatment plan by taking into account the target region's motion.

Multi-Layer Perceptron (MLP)
>   A feed-forward artificial neural network model consisting of multiple layers of perceptrons which, in turn, are controlled by nonlinear activation functions.

Multi-Leaf Collimator (MLC)
>   A device with multiple metallic leaves used to shape the beam of a radiotherapeutic device.

Multi-step linear methods (MULIN)
>   A prediction method based on a Taylor-like expansion of the prediction error.

Multiscale Autoregression (MAR)
>   MAR describes an algorithm which applies the ARMA method to the multiscale decomposition of a signal.

Normalised Least Mean Squares (nLMS)
>   An extension of the LMS algorithm, where the gradient is computed in a more robust, i.e., normalised, manner.

Object Coordinate System (OCS)
>   The coordinate system attached to a movable object (in contrast to the WCS).

Organ at Risk (OAR)
>   An organ which should be spared from radiation as much as possible.

Planning Target Volume (PTV)
>   The volume taken into account when planning irradiation.

Principal Component Analysis (PCA)
>   A way to transform possibly correlated variables to uncorrelated, so-called principal components.

Probability Density Function (PDF)
>   A function describing the likelihood for a random variable to occur at a given point.

Radial Basis Function (RBF)
>   A function $f : \mathbb{R}^n \mapsto \mathbb{R}$ whose value $f(\mathbf{x})$ only depends on the sample's distance

from the origin or a point c called *centre*, i.e., $f(\mathbf{x}) = f(\mathbf{y})$ for all $\|\mathbf{x} - \mathbf{c}\| = \|\mathbf{y} - \mathbf{c}\|$.

RAID
Redundant array of independent disks.

Real-time Position Management System (RPM)
A gating method.

Real-Time Respiratory Tracking (RTRT)
A radiation therapy device manufactured by Mitsubishi.

Recursive Least Squares (RLS)
An adaptive algorithm used to find coefficients which minimise a weighted linear least squares cost function.

Region of Interest (ROI)
A subset of an image used for processing, usually segmentation.

RF
Radio Frequency.

Root Mean Square (RMS)
The square root of the mean of the squares of a series of values.

Signal to noise ratio (SNR)
A measure to quantify how badly a signal has been corrupted by noise.

Singular Value Decomposition (SVD)
A special decomposition of a matrix $\mathbf{A}$ into a product of three matrices $\mathbf{U \Sigma V}^*$, where $\mathbf{U}$ and $\mathbf{V}$ are square unitary matrices and Σ is a real-valued matrix where only elements on its main diagonal can be non-zero.

SOMIT
Schonendes Operieren mit innovativer Technik, Gentle Surgery by Innovative Technology.

Sum of Squared Distances (SSD)
A metric used in image registration. It is computed as

$$\Sigma(A, B) = \sum_i \sum_j (\mathbf{A}(i, j) - \mathbf{B}(i, j))^2$$

and is used to determine the similarity of two images/volumes from the same imaging modality.

Support Vector Machine (SVM)
A supervised learning method which can classify data and recognise patterns. It can be used for statistical classification and regression analysis. It is a maximum margin classifier.

Support Vector Regression (SVR)
A regression method based on the concept of Support Vector Machines.

Support Vector Regression prediction (SVRpred)
A prediction method based on Support Vector Regression.

Synchronised Moving Aperture Radiation Therapy (SMART)
A method to synchronise the moving radiation beam formed by a DMLC to the tumour motion.

Transfer Control Protocol/Internet Protocol (TCP/IP)
    A family of network protocols used in the internet and local area networks.

U.S. Food and Drug Administration (FDA)
    An agency within the U.S. Department of Health and Human Services respon-
    sible for protecting the public health by assuring the safety, effectiveness, and
    security of human and veterinary drugs, vaccines and other biological products,
    medical devices, food supply, cosmetics, dietary supplements, and products that
    give off radiation.
Ultrasound (US)
    An imaging method using ultrasound.

Wavelet-based Multiscale Autoregression (wMAR)
    The application of the MAR algorithm to a wavelet decomposition of a signal.
Wavelet-based multiscale LMS prediction (wLMS)
    The extension of the $nLMS_2$ algorithm to a wavelet-based multiscale decompo-
    sition of an input signal.
World Coordinate System (WCS)
    A fixed reference coordinate system.

X-ray
    Electromagnetic radiation with a wavelength $\lambda \in [0.01, 10]$ nm.

Zero Error Prediction (ZEP)
    A prediction method by Accuray.